Discover a world of Tropical Fruit

A fully illustrated guide to over 100 nutritious, gluten free, exotic fruits

GLENN TANKARD

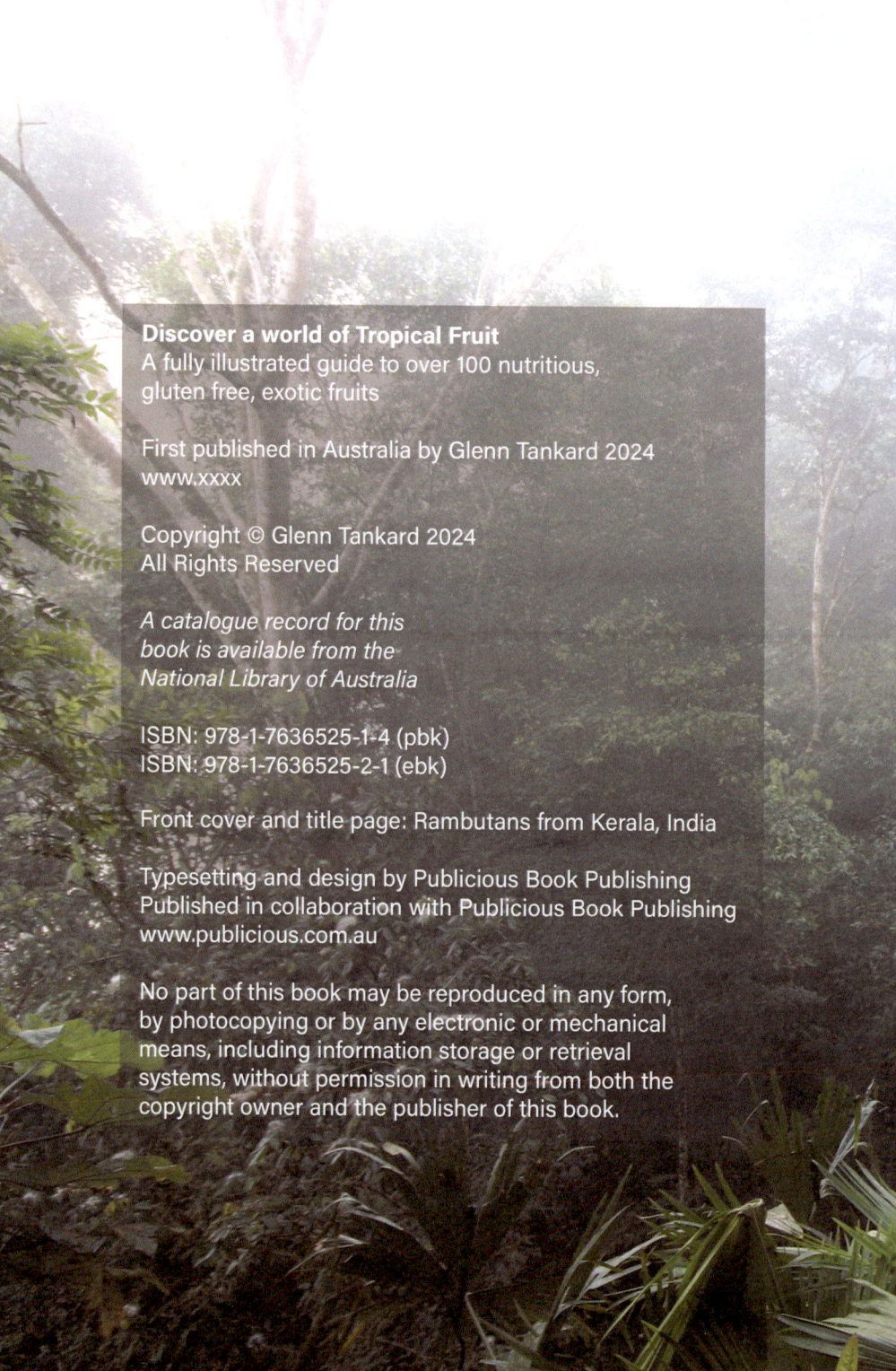

Discover a world of Tropical Fruit
A fully illustrated guide to over 100 nutritious, gluten free, exotic fruits

First published in Australia by Glenn Tankard 2024
www.xxxx

Copyright © Glenn Tankard 2024
All Rights Reserved

A catalogue record for this book is available from the National Library of Australia

ISBN: 978-1-7636525-1-4 (pbk)
ISBN: 978-1-7636525-2-1 (ebk)

Front cover and title page: Rambutans from Kerala, India

Typesetting and design by Publicious Book Publishing
Published in collaboration with Publicious Book Publishing
www.publicious.com.au

No part of this book may be reproduced in any form, by photocopying or by any electronic or mechanical means, including information storage or retrieval systems, without permission in writing from both the copyright owner and the publisher of this book.

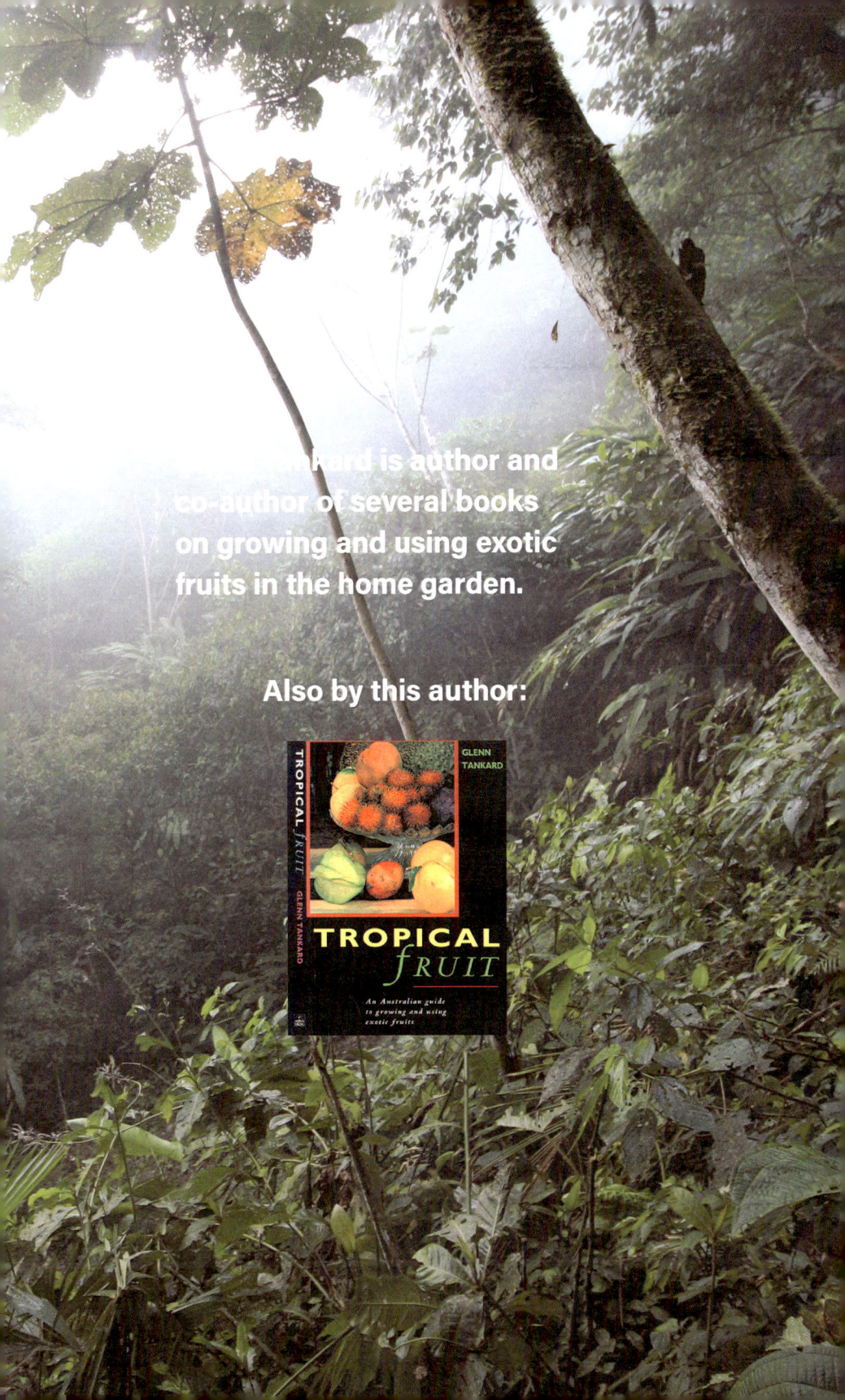

Glenn Tankard is author and co-author of several books on growing and using exotic fruits in the home garden.

Also by this author:

TROPICAL fruit
An Australian guide to growing and using exotic fruits
GLENN TANKARD

Contents

Introduction	
Abiu	1
Abyssinian dovyalis	2
Açai palm	3
Acerola	4
Ackee	5
Amazon tree grape	6
Ambarella	7
Araza	8
Atemoya	9
Avocado	10
Bael fruit	11
Bakupari	12
Barbados gooseberry	13
Bignay	14
Bilimbi	15
Black sapote	16
Borojo	17
Breadfruit	18
Bullocks heart	19
Burdekin plum	20
Caimito	21
Camu camu	22
Canistel	23
Carambola	24
Cashew fruit	25
Cecropia	26
Ceylon gooseberry	27
Cherimoya	28
Chinese jujube	29
Coco plum	30
Cocona	31
Coconut	32
Common guava	33

Cuban mangosteen	34
Dabai	35
Date	36
Downy rose cherry	37
Durian	38
Gamboge	39
Giant granadilla	40
Green sapote	41
Guavaberry	42
Herbert river cherry	43
Ilama	44
Imbe	45
Indian gooseberry	46
Inga	47
Jaboticaba	48
Jackfruit	49
Jelly palm	50
Kaffir plum	51
Karonda	52
Kei apple	53
Key lime	54
Kiwifruit	55
Kwai muk	56
Langsat	57
Lucuma	58
Mabolo	59
Madrono	60
Malay apple	61
Mamey sapote	62
Mangaba	63
Mango	64
Mangosteen	65
Maprang	66
Maqui berry	67
Matisia	68

Miracle fruit	69
Mountain soursop	70
Nance fruit	71
Naranjilla	72
Otaheite gooseberry	73
Panama berry	74
Papaya	75
Passionfruit	76
Peach palm	77
Persimmon	78
Pitaya	79
Pomegranate	80
Pomelo	81
Prickly pear	82
Pulasan	83
Rambai	84
Rambutan	85
Red mombin	86
Rollinia	87
Santol	88
Sapodilla	89
Sea grape	90
Seville orange	91
Soncoya	92
Soursop	93
Spanish lime	94
Strawberry guava	95
Sugar apple	96
Tamarillo	97
Umbu	98
Velvet Tamarind	99
Wampee	100
Yellow mombin	101
Photo Credits	102

Introduction

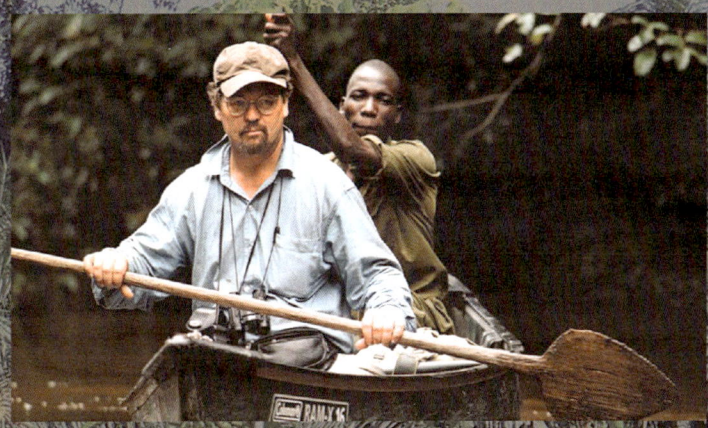

Rare fruit plant and seed hunter Alan Carle (botanicalark.com)

They journey to remote and often wild destinations in search of a strange new taste, a strange new fruit. From the upper reaches of the Amazon River in tropical Peru and Brazil, to the Incan territories high up in the Andes mountains. From the rainforests of the Western Ghats in India to the jungles of Papua New Guinea, Sarawak and Sabah. From the swamps of Thailand to the island paradise of Bali. They race against time, progress and the continual destruction of the wilderness areas of the world. They often return with the seeds of exciting new species. They are the plant hunters and seed collectors.

Currently with international travel more accessible we are moving around the globe far more readily than we were a few years ago. We visit tropical and subtropical destinations where we are likely to see and try exotic fruit in local markets, restaurants and even on excursions into the country. Even at home we now have access to a wider range of new and often strange fruits. Some are sweeter than others and are eaten fresh either alone or in salads. We call these "dessert" fruits. Other fruits are more tart or acidic and are more suitable for food preparations such as juices, jams, and ices. Then there are the savoury fruits that are used as we would vegetables.

This fully illustrated book serves as a handy guide to over 100 tropical fruits from all over the world. From the more common to the rarer fruit species. Discover exotic fruits from the Amazon such as the delicious, yellow skinned abiu, the camu camu absolutely packed with vitamin C, or the unusual, yellow-skinned custard apple known as rollinia. From the rainforests of Indonesia comes the durian, "King of tropical fruit", and Malaysia is home to the irresistible mangosteen, the "Queen of tropical fruits". These are just a few examples of the rare fruit species saved from extinction as a result of the continuing destruction of the world's rainforests.

The book lists each fruit's common name, botanical name, their native habitat, description, culinary use, nutritional value and any interesting facts and folklore. Come along on a discovery tour of the tropical fruits of the world.

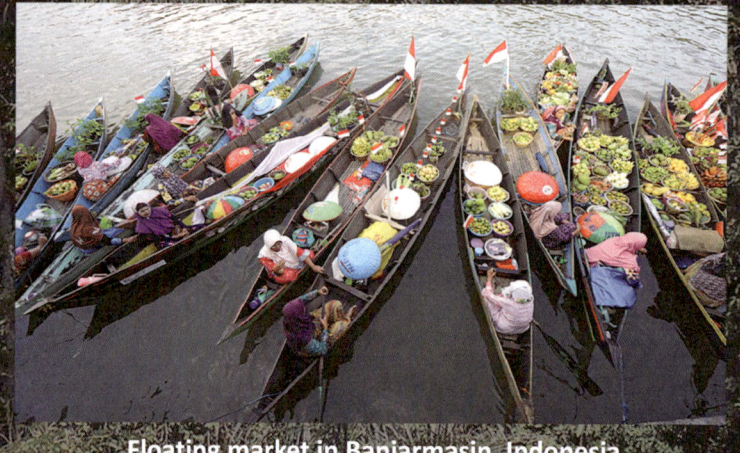

Floating market in Banjarmasin, Indonesia

Abiu
Pouteria caimito

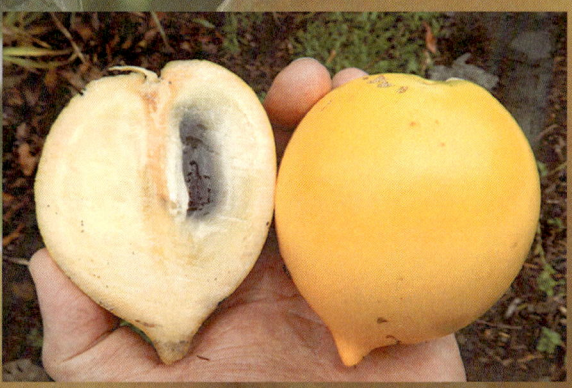

Other names
Caimito, yellow star apple, star apple, abio, caminito amarillo (Colombia), madura verde (Colombia), luma (Ecuador) cauje (Ecuador), temare (Venezuela), abieiro (Portugal), kepi (Bolivia), alasa (Ghana).

Native habitat
The abiu is home to the humid forests of the western Amazon, its native range extends across large swathes of Peru and Brazil.

Description
Abiu fruit vary from round to oval shape, and are pointed at the bottom. Ripe fruits have a smooth, bright yellow skin. Inside is a pale, white, translucent pulp with a creamy, jelly-like texture and a wonderful sweet caramel taste. There are 1-4 ovate, brown seeds which have some pulp attached and are easily removed.

Culinary Use
The fruits should be fully ripe to avoid the sticky white latex. Pulp is easily scooped out with a spoon. It is often just eaten out of hand but also goes well used in ice cream. Abius are harvested when fruits turn bright yellow and become fully ripe in 1-3 days in the fruit bowl. Harvested fruit has a shelf life of 7-14 days at 10°C.

Nutritional value
The fruit is rich in vitamins and minerals. It contains thiamine, riboflavin, niacin, vitamin C, calcium and iron.

Interesting facts and folklore
In Brazil the pulp is eaten to ease coughs and bronchitis. In Amazonia, abiu fruits are cultivated and sold in local markets.

Abyssinian dovyalis
Dovyalis abyssinica

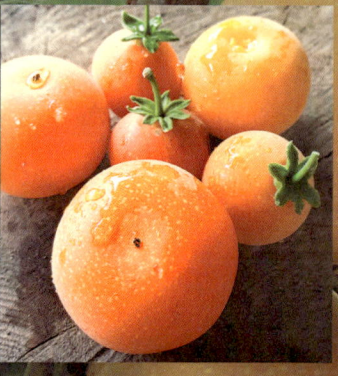

Other names
Koshim (Amargna), ankakute (Oromiffa), ongolatz (Somalgna), aihada (Tigrigna), Abyssinian gooseberry, koshum, mukambura.

Native habitat
It's a fruiting shrub or small tree originating in East Africa in the highland areas of Ethiopia, Eritrea, Somalia, Kenya, Tanzania and Malawi. Its natural habitat is highland forest 600- 1,800 metres above sea level. It is found in rainforest to dry evergreen forest with rocky limestone slopes.

Description
The small, round, orange fruit has thin, tender, velvety skins and a very juicy flesh with some small flattish white seeds. Ripe fruit has an acid to sub-acid flavour with a strong aroma and apricot flavoured flesh. Fruits are green when young ripening to orange-yellow and resemble miniature apricots covered in tiny white dots. They are harvested when firm, softening quickly.

Culinary Use
The fruit is usually too sour to be eaten fresh out-of-hand. They are mostly made into jam, syrup, juices, wine or dried like apricots. Just peel the tough skin and boil the pulp. Strain it, then boil it with equal parts sugar.

Nutritional value
The fruit pulp is high in vitamin C, is a good source of fibre, iron and phosphorus. They also contain small amounts of B-complex vitamins.

Interesting facts and folklore
The stems and branches are covered in grey-brown bark. They have strong, straight spines useful as a hedge to deter intruders or burglars.

Açai palm
Euterpe oleracea

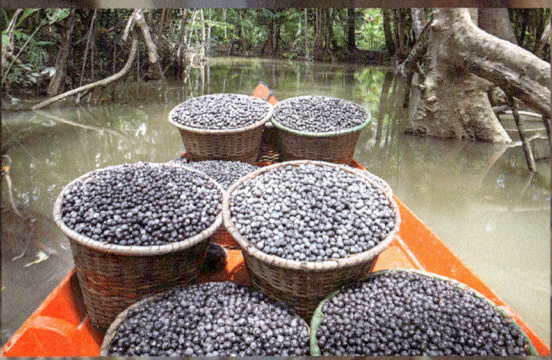

Other names
Açaí (Aa-sah-EE) Palm, Assai Palm, Acai Palma, Cabbage Palm, Pina Palm.

Native habitat
Açai palms form dense stands in the swampy floodplains and riverbanks on the Amazon lowlands in eastern Brazil. It's natural habitat is the Amazon river basin and estuary.

Description
The fruit is small (1.5 cm), round, and black-purple in colour. Each fruit contains a large seed which accounts for most of its volume. The thin outer coating of flesh is the berry and is what we consume as a juice, pulp or powder. Berries are harvested when they ripen from green to a deep purple. They have a flavour described as a blend of chocolate and berries, with a little metallic aftertaste.

Culinary Use
Açai berries spoil quickly after picking due to their high fat content so they are best eaten fresh out of hand. Local tribes use the pulp of the fresh fruit in a variety of drinks, including wine. Most açai is now destined for export, the fruit pulp is dried and powdered as a popular dietary supplement.

Nutritional value
Acai berries are rich in fatty acids, especially oleic, palmitic and linoleic acids. They are rich in antioxidants, vitamins, and minerals. They have a high anthocyanin pigment content that is a potent antioxidant and anti-inflammatory.

Interesting facts and folklore
Due to their popularity, hearts of palm have decimated many palm tree populations in parts of South America, including the acai palm.

Acerola
Malpighia emarginata

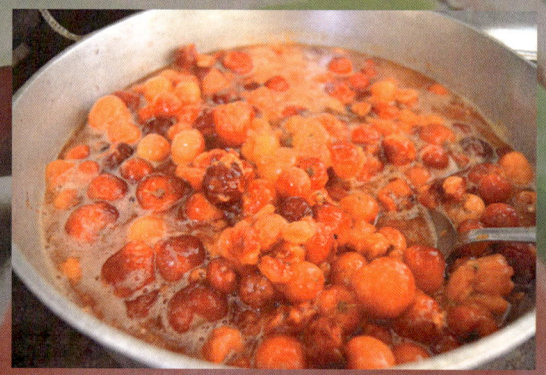

Other names
Barbados cherry, West Indian cherry, Puerto Rican cherry, Antilles cherry, cereso, cereza, cerisier, semeruco, guarani cherry.

Native habitat
Acerola is a tropical shrub that thrives in warm, lowland frost free climates and is native to the Caribbean islands, Central and South America, southern Mexico, Puerto Rico.

Description
The fruits are tri- lobed (1-3 cm), bright red berries, very juicy and aromatic, with a taste that's sweet to sour depending upon ripeness. They have glossy, red to crimson, thin skins and taste similar to apples. There are 3 triangular seeds. They grow in pairs or groups of threes.

Culinary Use
As well as being eaten out of hand, they can also be stewed, made into juices, sauces, jellies, jams, wines or purees. They have a shelf life of only 2-3 days. Normally they are boiled, sweetened, strained and served as a dessert fruit. The juice can be mixed with coconut water or pineapple juice. Toppings for ice cream are popular.

Nutritional value
It is a very rich source of vitamin C. It also contains many minerals and other vitamins, including beta-carotene, lutein, thiamine, riboflavin, niacin, pyridoxine, folic acid, and pantothenic acid. A glass of acerola juice contains as much ascorbic acid as 14 litres of orange juice.

Interesting facts and folklore
Extracts of the fruit are used as antioxidants in formulations against skin inflammation and redness. Acerola berries are considered beneficial against liver problems, diarrhoea, dysentery, coughs and colds.

Ackee
Blighia sapida

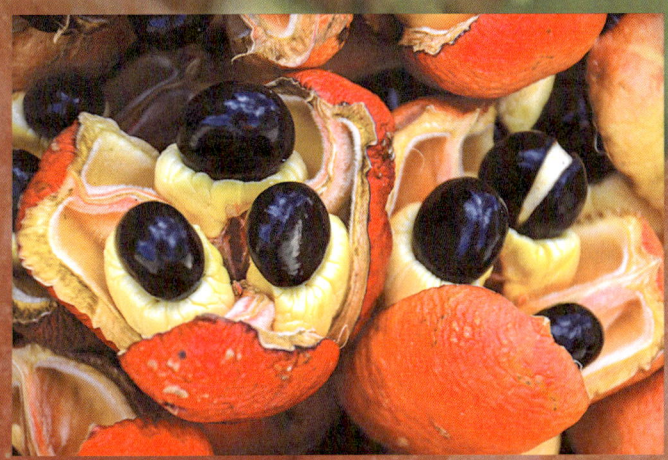

Other names
Ackee apple, akee, seso vegetal, acki.

Native habitat
Akee is native to West Africa along the Gold Coast and Ivory Coast.

Description
Fruits are tri-lobed pear-shaped capsules. They mature from green to scarlet-red in 7-8 weeks, splitting open to reveal 3 large shiny black seeds and fleshy creamy-yellow aril. Aril is edible when fully ripe and the fruit splits open.

Culinary Use
Fully-ripe fresh aril is edible when fruits split open. Aril has nutty flavour and is eaten in Jamaica as part of the national dish, or canned. eaten raw when fully ripe. The fleshy arils surrounding the seeds are firm and oily, with a nutty flavour. Flesh can also be curried, used in soups, stews, soufflés.

Nutritional value
Ackees provide a large percentage of our daily copper requirement. They are rich in potassium, magnesium, calcium, sodium and zinc.

Interesting facts and folklore
The genus *Blighia* is named after Captain Wiliam Bligh (of 'Mutiny on the Bounty' fame), who saw the fruit in Jamaica and took it to England in 1793. Its Jamaica's national fruit and when eaten with salt-fish it is called the national dish. Jamaicans love ackee and the country is often referred to as the "Big Ackee". The ripe aril is consumed to lower fever and treat dysentery.

Amazon tree grape
Pourouma cecropiifolia

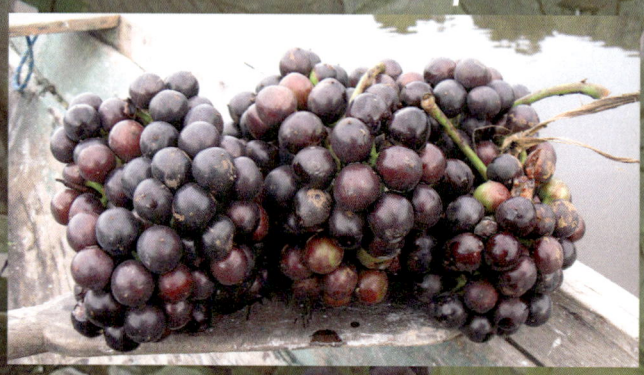

Other names
Amazon grape, Uvilla (which translates to "little grape" in Spanish), caimaron, curcura, cucura, peruma, uva.

Native habitat
The Amazon tree grape is native to tropical South America. Its home is in the western Amazon basin in the foothills of the Andes. In northern Bolivia, western Brazil, south-eastern Colombia, eastern Ecuador, eastern Peru, and southern Venezuela.

Description
The fruit is round (up to 4cm), purple when ripe, resembling grapes in flavour. The skin is rough, fibrous, inedible but is easily peeled. The white pulp is sweet, succulent and juicy. There is a single hard, oval-shaped seed. They grow in bunches of up to 20 fruits and have a short shelf life.

Culinary Use
The grapes are eaten fresh and made into jams and jellies. Fermented fruit is used to make wine. Toasted seeds are used as a coffee substitute.

Nutritional value
The tree grape contains vitamins A and C, is high in sugars and contains minerals such as potassium, phosphorus, magnesium and calcium. The peel is high in anthocyanins.

Interesting facts and folklore
In 1596 explorer Gonzalo Quesada came across plantations of the tree grape in "gardens of vegetables and fruit plants" in the eastern Llanos of Colombia. He said the species was cultivated and most likely domesticated since the pre-Columbian period. The Ticuna people today have large plantations around their villages in the Tabatinga district in Brazil, Leticia in Colombia and Iquitos in Peru.

Ambarella
Spondias dulcis

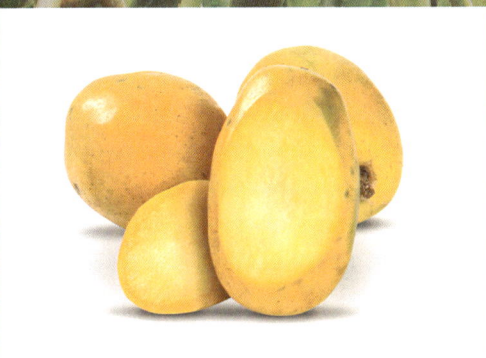

Other names
Golden apple, June plum, Otaheite apple, Pommecythere or Cythere, Kedondong, Great Hog Plum, Yellow Plum, Hog plum, Jew plum, Polynesian plum, Tahitian quince, cajamanga.

Native habitat
Ambarella is native to the South Pacific islands, from Melanesia through to Polynesia. Its habitat is in dry or secondary forests from sea-level to 500 metres. Trees thrive in subtropical and tropical environments.

Description
Ambarella are oval fruits, 6–9 cm long, and are borne in bunches of 12 or more on a long stalk. Over a period of several weeks, the fruit falls to the ground while still green and hard, then turns golden-yellow as they ripen. They have a firm, orange-yellow, juicy pulp that is crunchy and tastes like a mix of mango and pineapple. They have a single, large spiny seed.

Culinary Use
Ripe fruit can be eaten fresh out-of-hand but are mostly stewed and made into preserves, such as jams and chutneys. They are made into fruit sauces for cheesecakes, ice cream and yoghurts. In Indonesia they steam the fruit to accompany salted fish and rice.

Nutritional value
Vitamins B1,C, and A, calcium and phosphorus.

Interesting facts and folklore
The seed has sharp spines that can be painful when eating the fruit. The grated fruit mixed in water has diuretic properties and is used to treat high blood pressure. Bangkok's original name was "Bang Makok," which translates into "river town where Kedondongs grow."

Araza
Eugenia stipitata

Other names
Araçá-boi, Amazonian pear, arasa, membrillo.

Native habitat
Araza is native to the Amazon rainforest in Brazil, Colombia and Ecuador. It's habitat is as an understory plant in the humid lowland rainforests, and can be found above the floodplains growing in highly leached soils.

Description
Fruits are round, the pale green, thin velvety skins turning to bright yellow when ripe. Fruits are juicy, aromatic, and very acidic when eaten freshly picked. Their pH is similar to that of lemons and rarely eaten raw. Fruits have 8-12 seeds within the thick, juicy, golden yellow flesh. Ripe fruits last up to 5 days at room temperature.

Culinary Use
Once the seeds are removed from the yellowish pulp it is commonly processed into juices, nectars, marmalades, ice-creams, hot sauce and alcohol.

Nutritional value
Araza has vitamin C, B1, and A.

Interesting facts and folklore
Araza is high in vitamin C, double the amount of an orange. It is a semi-domesticated plant of the western Amazon basin. As a member of the Myrtle family, araza is related to guava, grumichama and jaboticaba. Araza are a rare species and not commonly seen outside their natural habitat.

Atemoya

Annona squamosa × *Annona cherimola*

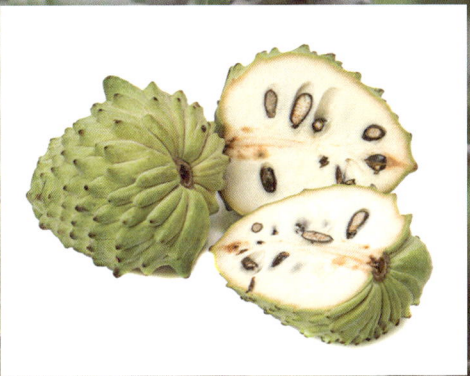

Other names
Pineapple sugar apple, anón, chirimorinon, custard apple.

Native habitat
The atemoya is a man-made hybrid between the cherimoya, native to the Andes mountains, and the sugar apple, a native of the Caribbean.

Description
Atemoya fruit are heart-shaped or rounded, with pale-green, easily bruised, bumpy skin and weigh up to 2kg. Near the stem, the skin is bumpy as it is in the sugar-apple, but becomes smoother like the cherimoya on the bottom. Their creamy-white, juicy flesh has an agreeable blend of mild acidity and sweetness. It is very juicy and smooth, with a taste resembling banana, pineapple, strawberry and some vanilla from its sugar apple parent. Many toxic, black seeds are found throughout the flesh.

Culinary Use
Serve chilled and simply cut in half and scoop out the flesh from the shell, discarding the seeds. The pulp may be added to fruit salads or desserts. Fully ripened fruit can be refrigerated for one to two days.

Nutritional value
Atemoyas are high in vitamin C and B1, potassium and fibre. They also have magnesium, iron, zinc, and phosphorus.

Interesting facts and folklore
The initial hybridisation was made in 1908 by P.J. Wester. The common name atemoya, is a combination of ate, an old Mexican name for sugar apple, and "moya" from cherimoya.

Avocado
Persea americano

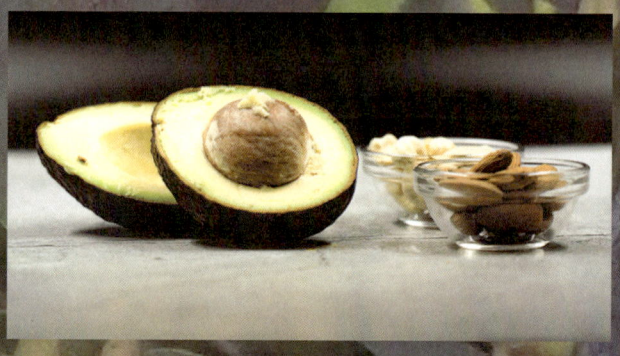

Other names
Alligator pear (due to its bumpy green skin and pear shape), avocado pear.

Native habitat
Avocados originated in the highlands from Mexico and Guatemala. The native habitat is a moist, tropical, evergreen or mountain forest, and on the lower slopes of rainforests, with very well-drained soils.

Description
The avocado is botanically a large berry containing a single large seed. It has a smooth, buttery, golden-green flesh when ripe. Depending on the cultivar, avocados have green, brown, purplish, or black skin, and may be pear-shaped, egg-shaped, or spherical.

Culinary Use:
Avocado is used in both savoury and sweet dishes. It is the base for the Mexican dip known as guacamole and is used as a spread on corn tortillas or toast. In their homeland Mexico and Central America they are served mixed with white rice, in soups, salads, or on the side of meat dishes.

Nutritional value
Avocado is a rich source of several B vitamins and vitamin K. It has moderate amounts of vitamin C, vitamin E, and potassium. They also contain phytosterols and carotenoids. Its energy value mainly comes from monounsaturated fat.

Interesting facts and folklore
There are two flowering types of avocado. A-type flowers open as female on the morning of the first day and close in late morning and then they open as male in the afternoon of the second day. B varieties have an overlapping flowering pattern to this so you need to plant both types to ensure a good fruit set.

Bael fruit
Aegle marmelos

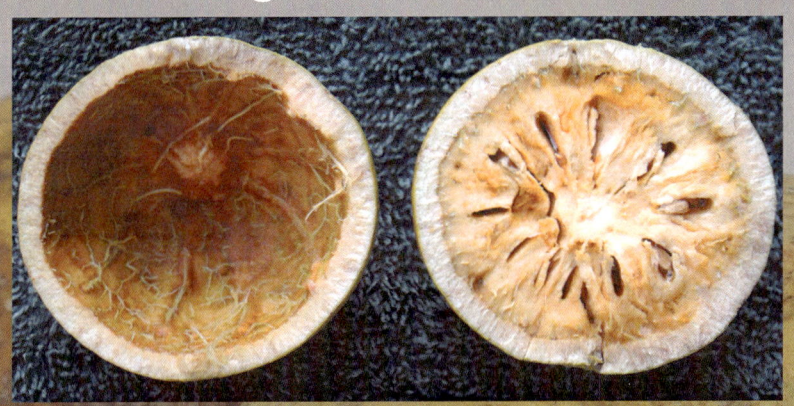

Other names
Bengal quince, bilva, golden apple, Japanese bitter orange, stone apple or wood apple.

Native habitat
Bael fruit is native to the Indian subcontinent and Southeast Asia. Trees thrive in warm and humid climates, preferring well-drained soil. They are found growing wild in forests and along riverbanks at elevations up to 1,200 metres.

Description
Bael fruit is round to pear-shaped with a hard yellowish- brown skin. The fibrous pulp is soft and aromatic ranging from pale-orange to reddish, filled with small, flat seeds. The flavour is a blend of sweet, tangy, and bitter.

Culinary Use
Bael fruits are suitable for fresh, cooked, or dried preparations. They are used to make beverages like sherbets and juices, jams, chutneys, and desserts. They can be simmered into syrup, cooked into chutney, and added to puddings. Fruits are juiced for cold drinks and tea, often mixed with citrus, water, and sugar. Stored whole in the refrigerator, they can keep up to 2 weeks.

Nutritional value
It's rich in vitamin C, A and B. It also has calcium, iron and potassium and provides fibre.

Interesting facts and folklore
Bael fruits are deeply intertwined with Hindu worship, particularly Lord Shiva. The tree's leaves symbolise Shiva's trident and are used in temple rituals to cleanse sins.

Bakupari
Garcinia gardneriana

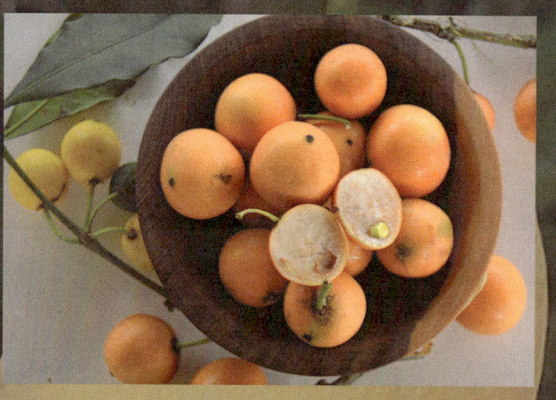

Other names
Bacupari, achacha, achachai, guapomo, achuchaira (honey kiss in Guarani).

Native habitat
Native to Brazil, Bolivia, Peru, Ecuador, Venezuela. It grows in rainforests, along river banks where it can access water.

Description
Bakupari fruit is a berry with a smooth and hard thick skin. It changes from a bluish-green to orange-reddish colour as it ripens. The flavour is similar to feijoa and citrus, sweet and refreshing. The leathery rind encloses a juicy, white, aromatic pulp with a large brown seed.

Culinary Use
The fruit are eaten fresh out-of-hand by cracking the leathery rind with the fingernail, then peeling it to access the pulp, which is usually sucked away from the seed in the mouth. The pulp is used as a flavouring for ice cream, popsicles, jam, jellies and even liquor.

Nutritional value
Bakupari has large amounts of xanthones, benzophenones, phloroglucinols, and bioflavonoids.

Interesting facts and folklore
Each year in December, in the city of Santa Cruz de la Sierra, in Bolivia a festival is held to honour the fruit harvest. The fruit's name bakuparí comes from the Tupi-Guarani language and means "hedge fruit" due to its horizontal branching habit.

Barbados gooseberry
Pereskia aculeata

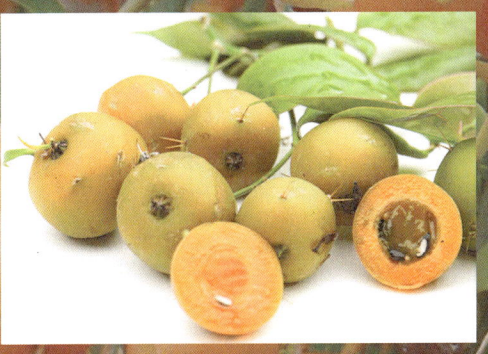

Other names
Blade-apple cactus, leaf cactus, rose cactus, lemonvine, West Indian gooseberry, ora-pro-nobis.

Native habitat
It is native to Central America, the Caribbean and South America. In the Antilles, Panama and Colombia. It grows wild as a primitive climbing cactus along stream banks, rainforest and dry, open forest.

Description
The light yellow, orange or red fruit is a small (1-2 cm) rounded to oval shaped berry, containing several small, flat, brown or black soft seeds. They resemble a gooseberry in appearance and have smooth, leathery skins. They have a very pleasant acid to tart taste.

Culinary Use
Fruits are eaten fresh, stewed or preserved with sugar, or made into jams and jellies. Pectin needs to be added to make jam and jelly since the fruit is low in it and doesn't gel.

Nutritional value
Barbados gooseberry fruit have a high vitamin A and medium calcium content.

Interesting facts and folklore
The Barbados gooseberry is a scrambling shrubby cactus or vine in the Cactaceae family. Capuchin and brown howler monkeys feed on the fruits, and in some regions of Brazil are its main dispersers. It is a declared weed in many states as it chokes out large trees. The flea-beetle, *Phenrica guerini* has been used as a control measure with some limited success in South African plots. The leaves which are very high in protein are an important vegetable food in parts of rural Brazil.

Bignay
Antidesma bunius

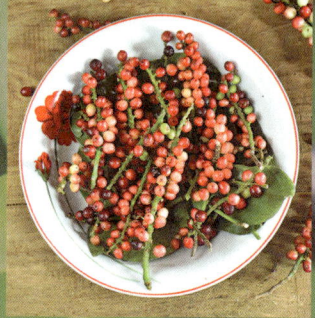

Other names
Bungay, Chinese laurel, Queensland cherry, wild cherry, current tree, salamander tree.

Native habitat
Bignay is native to a large region from Southeast Asia, Melanesia, to northern Australia. The trees thrive in hot, humid tropical environments and can be found in wet evergreen forests, dipterocarp forests, river banks, forest edges, roadsides, and even semi-cultivated areas.

Description
Bignay, also known as wild cherry, is a small, round or slightly oval shaped fruit. When fully ripe, they range from deep red to almost black, with a glossy thin skin. Bignay fruits have a sweet and tart flavour, resembling a mix of cherry, grape and cranberry. Each fruit contains one to three small edible seeds. Ripe fruits have a pleasant fruity aroma. They grow in clusters, turning deep purplish-red as they ripen. They have a sour taste when unripe, but they sweeten with a pleasant tartness at maturity.

Culinary Use
Bignay fruits are used to make refreshing beverages like juices, wines, and sherbets. They are suitable for making jams, jellies, and preserves, offering a unique sweet and tart flavour. The fruits can be cooked into sauces or chutneys. They give a tang to desserts such as pies, tarts, cakes, and ice creams.

Nutritional value
Bignay fruit is rich in vitamin C and vitamin A and also contain calcium, iron, phosphorus and anthocyanins.

Interesting facts and folklore
In the Philippines bignay wine represents unity, joy, community, tradition, and national pride.

Bilimbi
Averrhoa bilimbi

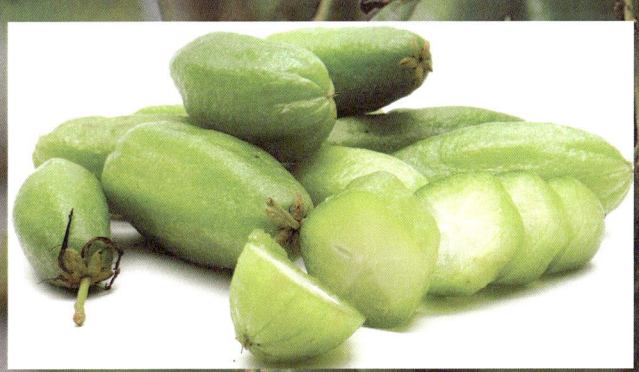

Other names
Tree cucumber, pickle tree, billing-billing, belimbing, bullhorn, blimbing, balimbing, taling pling, kaling pling, pias, camias, khe tay.

Native habitat
Bilimbi is native to the Maluku islands of Indonesia. It is also found in tropical regions of India and other parts of South Asia. Bilimbi trees thrive in warm, humid climates with well-drained soil, typically growing in tropical rainforests, gardens, and orchards.

Description
Bilimbi fruits are small and slender, resembling a small cucumber. Fruits ripen from green to greenish-yellow to almost white in cases, with a smooth delicate skin that is readily bruised. Their flavour is sour, similar to lemon. Several small seeds are present but usually not eaten. When sliced in half the fruit has a five pointed star in the centre like carambola.

Culinary Use
Bilimbi fruit has a tangy and sour taste that is best suited to cooked dishes. It can be eaten raw with added salt, sugar, or spices. The fruit is commonly used to make juices, syrups, and vinegar. It is suitable for preserves, chutneys, pickles, jams, and sauces.

Nutritional value
Bilimbi fruits are rich in nutrients such as vitamin C, vitamin A, potassium, and minerals calcium, magnesium, iron, zinc, manganese, copper, and phosphorus.

Interesting facts and folklore
Bilimbi is added to curries, soups, dals, and fish dishes for its sourness. Bilimbi is used in traditional medicine for coughs, fevers, and skin health.

Black sapote
Diospyros nigra

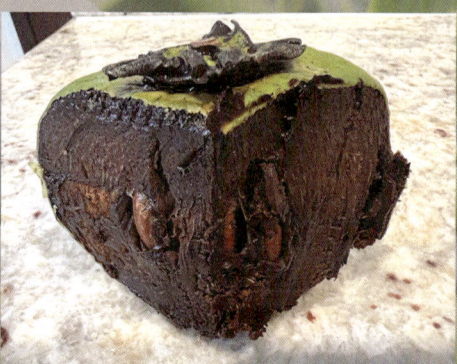

Other names
Chocolate pudding fruit, ironwood, black persimmon, zapote negro (in Spanish), mamey sapote, chocolate fruit, chocolate persimmon, sapote prieto.

Native habitat
Indigenous to Mexico, Central America, and Colombia.

Description
Black sapote fruits are olive green, round (5-10 cm) with a dark brown to black soft pulp resembling chocolate pudding. It has a very rich, sweet flavour. Harvested green fruit remains quite firm for 3-6 days then ripen marshmallow soft, almost miraculously, overnight. Fruits contain up to 12 smooth, brown seeds.

Culinary Use
It makes delicious ice cream and milkshakes. It also adds flavour and texture in mousses, cakes, bread and preserves. For a simple treat mix the pulp with lemon juice and yoghurt. Cut fruits in half and cover the flesh with passionfruit. Mash the pulp with orange juice or brandy and serve with fresh cream. It is also nice mixed with wine, sugar and cinnamon. To open the fruit, cut it around the midline and twist the two halves to pull it apart. Use a sharp pointed knife to remove seeds and spoon out the delicious pulp.

Nutritional value
Excellent source of vitamin C, about four times as much as an orange and 100g is 6 times the daily value. It also has calcium and phosphorus.

Interesting facts and folklore
Diospyros means divine fruit and is derived from the Greek words "dios" and "pyron", and can mean food of the gods, God's pear, wheat of Zeus or Jove's fire.

Borojo
Alibertia patinoi

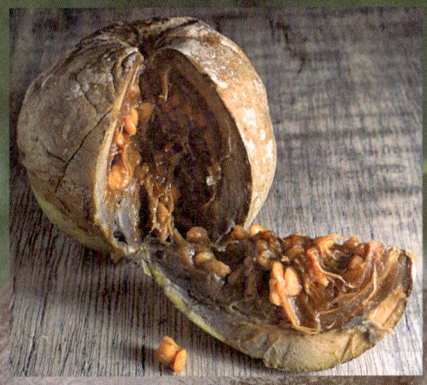

Other names
Colombian sweetberry, Borojoa patinoi.

Native habitat
Borojo is native to the humid tropical rainforests of the Chocó region in Colombia and also found in parts of Panama and Ecuador. It is native to some of the wettest regions of the lowland Amazon rainforest usually at elevations up to 700 metres.

Description
Borojo is a green to brown, round fruit with a sweet, tangy, acid and aromatic flavour. The texture of the brown flesh is dense, sticky brown, smooth and melting. The flavour has been compared to a plum with vanilla and tamarind overtones. The fruit can grow up to 1kg in weight. They may take up to 12 months to ripen. When ripe they turn brown and fall off the tree.

Culinary Use
Borojo fruit can be eaten raw or made into preserves, juices and jellies. The fruit pulp is used to prepare a juice (jugo del amor), sauce, marmalades, wine and various flavourings.

Nutritional value
Borojo has high levels of protein, vitamins B and C, calcium and iron and very high levels of phosphorus.

Interesting facts and folklore
Borojó is an Emberá word meaning head-shaped fruit, a dialect spoken by people in northwestern Colombia and southeastern Panama. Borojo juice is used in traditional medicines to treat bronchitis and hypertension. It also has supposed aphrodisiac and energising effects.

Breadfruit
Artocarpus altillis

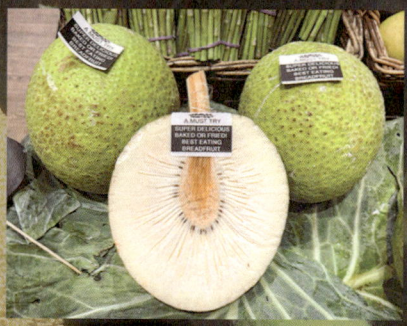

Other names
Fruta de pan, sa-ke, ulu, tree potato, suku, sukun, rimas, panapen, pan de ano, mazapan, arbor de pan, pao de massa, fruta pao.

Native habitat
Breadfruit is native to Southeast Asia and the Pacific Islands. It thrives in warm and wet, tropical climates and flourishes in coastal areas, lowland forests, and well-drained soils.

Description
Breadfruit, is a large, round to oval shaped fruit with a yellowish-green or yellow skin when mature. It has a tough skin with spiky bumps. It has creamy white to pale yellow starchy flesh with a mildly sweet taste when cooked. Fruit usually has small, edible seeds. It is cooked before eating and has a sweet, fragrant aroma reminiscent of freshly baked bread.

Culinary Use
Breadfruit is a staple food in tropical regions and can be boiled, roasted, fried, steamed, or baked. Its starchy flesh, similar to potatoes, is enjoyed in various dishes when young and green, including as a base for savoury meals. When ripe, breadfruit's sweetness increases, making it suitable for desserts like pancakes, pies, or puddings, or even for raw consumption.

Nutritional value
Breadfruit is rich in complex carbohydrates and high in dietary fibre. It contains vitamin A, B andC, potassium, magnesium, iron, phosphorus, and niacin.

Interesting facts and folklore
HMS Bounty had left England in 1787 on a mission to collect and transport breadfruit plants from Tahiti to the West Indies. Relations between Bligh and his crew deteriorated a few weeks after leaving Tahiti and the famous "Mutiny on the Bounty" transpired.

Bullocks heart
Annona reticulata

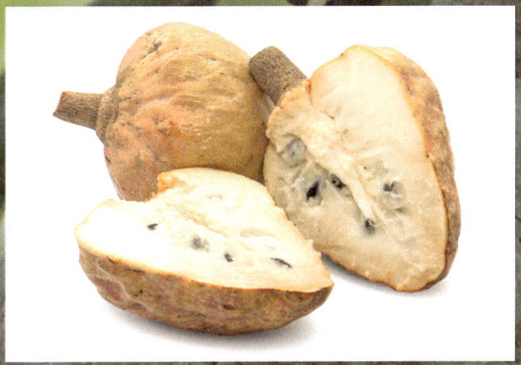

Other names
Mexican custard apple, ox-heart, wild sweetsop, binuwa, Corazón, sweetsop, anona corazon, Jamaica apple, maman netted custard apple.

Native habitat
Native to the West Indies and Central America, growing from sea level to 1500 metres in the tropics where there is a wet/dry climate.

Description
Fruits are edible but the quality varies considerably between varieties. Some are lacking in flavour and have a hard, sometimes bland and repulsive taste. Better types have a sweet, creamy, white or pale yellow flesh. Fruits are round, heart shaped, spherical or oblong. They are rough and yellow in colour which changes to yellowish red on ripening. They are sweet, astringent. The fruit lacks flavour and doesn't taste as good as cherimoya or atemoya .The flesh, like the other Annonas, is pulpy and contains numerous brown seeds.

Culinary Use
As the fruit varies considerably in quality, some are eaten raw but mostly they are used in preserves, drinks, ice cream, and puddings . In India the pulp is cooked into a sauce.

Nutritional value
Rich vitamin C, vitamin B6, magnesium, and Iron.

Interesting facts and folklore
Traditionally bullocks heart has been used to treat epilepsy, dysentery, heart problems and worm infestations. It also was good for constipation, bleeding, bacterial infections, fevers, ulcers and as insecticide. Tree leaves have been used for helminthiasis treatment. Bark from the tree roots has been used to relieve toothaches.

Burdekin plum
Pleiogynium timorense

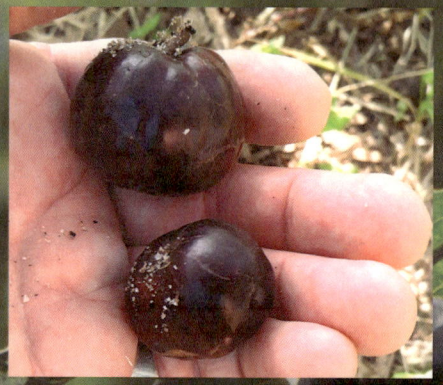

Other names
Sweet plum, Tulip plum, Guybalum (Djabugay language).

Native habitat
Burdekin plum is native to Malesia, Australia and the Pacific Islands, It grows in rainforest and wet-dry monsoon forest at elevations from sea level to 1,000 m. It grows naturally on sand dunes behind mangroves and in dry sub-coastal regions.

Description
Burdekin plums are plump, acidic fruits that are only edible when fully ripe. They are round, black in colour and contain a large stone. Flesh is mostly plum-coloured and tart however there are greenish-white varieties with a milder, sweet-tart flavour.

Culinary Use
The plums may be eaten raw, cooked into jams, jellies and preserves or fermented into wine. They are rather acidic freshly harvested off the tree and need to be stored for a few days. The flavour is of mango, pears, and apricot. The skins can be dried and used to flavour milkshakes and smoothies, or brewed to make tea.The Burdekin plum is often used to make pies, cakes, muffins and breads. The pulp also makes a nice topping for ice cream.

Nutritional value
Burdekin plums contain vitamin C, minerals, and dietary fibre, and nearly 5 times the antioxidant content of blueberries. They are also a good source of vitamin A.

Interesting facts and folklore
Aborigines were known to bury the fruit to help them ripen. The plums are eaten by cassowaries and great bowerbirds.

Caimito
Chrysophyllum cainito

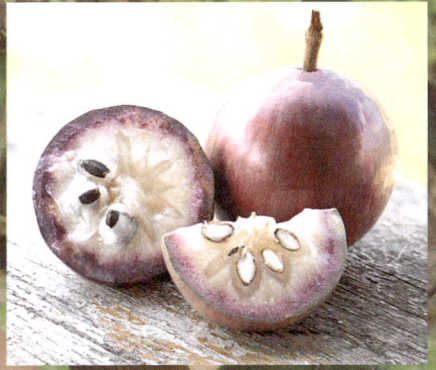

Other names
Star apple, cainito, golden-leaf star apple, abiu amarillo, golden leaf tree, abiaba, milk fruit.

Native habitat
Caimito comes from the Caribbean, its native habitat extending across the chain of islands from Jamaica, through the Cayman Islands, Cuba and Hispaniola, to Puerto Rico.

Description
The ripe fruit is round (5-8 cm), has a purple skin and a radiating star pattern is visible in the pulp. The skin is rich in a sticky latex, and both it and the rind are not eaten. It is sweet and often served chilled. The flesh is white, soft, milky and sweet and typically has 6-11 seeds. Fruit does not fall when ripe and therefore must be harvested by hand when fully mature.

Culinary Use
Caimito fruit is eaten fresh, or in fruit salads and sorbets. If you cut the fruit transversely and then separate the two halves you'll find it's the easiest way to open them. The pulp then can be spooned out, leaving the inedible seed cells, the seeds themselves, and the fruit core.

Nutritional value
Caimito is nutritious, containing moderate amounts of calcium, phosphorus, ascorbic acid (vitamin C), and a good source of antioxidants.

Interesting facts and folklore
The genus name comes from the Greek *chrysos* meaning "gold" and *phyllon* meaning "leaf", as the leaf undersides are a beautiful golden colour and make for a wonderful specimen tree.

Camu camu
Myrciaria dubia

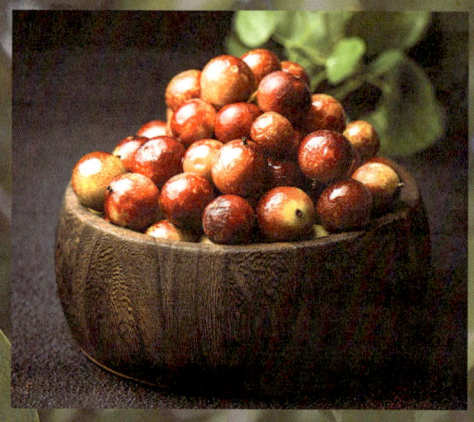

Other names
Cacari, camo camo, araçá-d'água, guayabo, guayabato.

Native habitat
Camu camu is native to the Amazonian lowlands of Colombia, Ecuador, Peru, Bolivia, and Brazil. In its native habitat it grows beside streams and lakes and in swamps.

Description
Camu camu fruit is maroon or purple-black when fully ripe, around 2.5-3 cm in diameter, with either sweet or acidic flesh. The berries are red to purple when ripe and have a pink pulp with 1-4 kidney-shaped seeds.

Culinary Use
The fruit juice or pulp is used to flavour other juices, ice creams, candy, and yoghurt. The juice can be very sour and usually needs to be diluted and sweetened. The berries, which are yellowish/red, tend to be very sour, which is why they are commonly ground into a powder like maqui berry and mixed with other foods. Now discovered and recognised as a superfood, , most camu camu fruits are sold as a powder and exported from their native lands.

Nutritional value
Absolutely loaded with vitamin C along with many other potent compounds like flavonoid antioxidants, including anthocyanins, ellagic acid and rutin.

Interesting facts and folklore
Camu camu contains 30 times more vitamin C compared to an orange. Acerola and acai are two better known superfoods however camu camu actually provides even more vitamin C than both.

Canistel
Pouteria campechiana

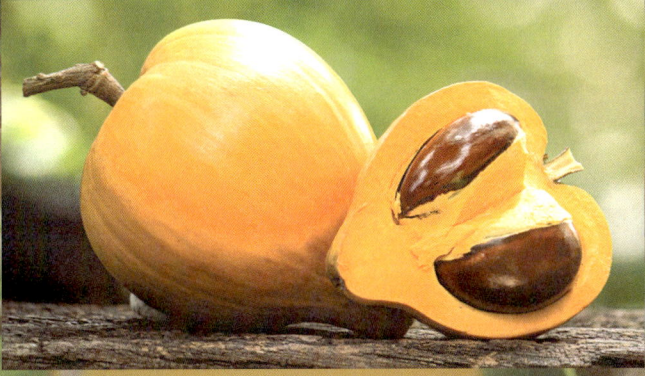

Other names
Eggfruit, yellow sapote, sapote amarillo, zapote borracho.

Native habitat
The canistel is native to Central America, from Panama, north to Mexico. The natural habitat is a moist or wet mixed forest, pine forests, often growing on limestone, at elevations from sea level to 1400 metres.

Description
Canistel fruit shape ranges from round to oval, with a pointed tip. The skin is thin, waxy, smooth, and green when unripe and bright yellow to orange when ripe. The pulp in better varieties is firm, smooth, creamy, and sweet and deep yellow when ripe. It is slightly dry with the consistency of a boiled egg. Canistel have up to 5 glossy, brown seeds. Like its relatives the mamey sapote and the sapodilla, the canistel has a flavour similar to pumpkin pie or roasted sweet potato.

Culinary Use
The fruit is commonly eaten fresh out of hand with a little salt and lemon juice added. The pulp is added to custards or made into eggnog-like milk drinks. The flesh can be dried and ground into a powder. Canistel pulp is used to make a smooth textured ice cream.

Nutritional value
Canistel is a good source of potassium, calcium and vitamins A and C.

Interesting facts and folklore
A latex extracted from the bark is used for making natural rubber. The scientific name campechiana is derived from the Mexican town of Campeche from which the trees are native.

Carambola
Averrhoa carambola

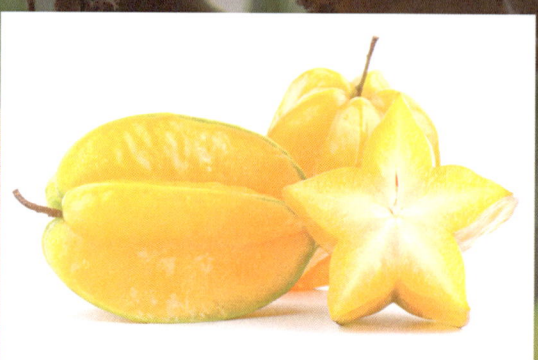

Other names
Star fruit, belimbing besi, belimbing manis, kembola, caramba, country gooseberry, kamrak.

Native habitat
Carambola is native to the Moluccas Islands in Malaysia, also known as the Spice Islands. It grows in humid forests and woodland on sandy loam in both tropical and subtropical regions.

Description
Carambola fruits are oblong in shape and mature from dark or light green to orangey-yellow, featuring 5 or 6 ribs and a star shape when sliced. They have a juicy, crisp yellow flesh that is sweet-tart when ripe and tastes similar to apple, pear or grape. The fruit's aroma is reminiscent of grapes or plums. The entire fruit, including the waxy skin and seeds, is edible.

Culinary Use
Fruit is eaten fresh, sliced, or juiced. They can be combined with apples, sugar, and cloves. Use sour unripe fruit for jams. Keep ripe, unwashed fruits refrigerated for up to a month or at room temp for two weeks.

Nutritional value:
Rich in carbohydrates and fibre, antioxidants, vitamins (A, C, B-complex) and minerals potassium and phosphorus.

Interesting facts and folklore
Carambolas' star shape makes them a popular decorative element when sliced for fruit punches or salads. Carambola is nicknamed star fruit for its five golden points that reveal a star shape when cut crosswise. The generic name *Averrhoa* is after Averroes (1126-98), the widely known Arab Philosopher of the time.

Cashew fruit
Anarcardium occidentale

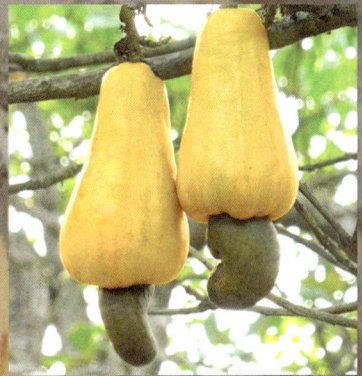

Other names
Cashew apple, cashew nut, Jagus, Gandaria, Gajus, Janggus, Jambu Gajus, Jambu Golok, Keterek, Terek, Jambu Bongkok caju, or Cajueiro.

Native habitat
North-eastern Brazil, typically growing in the dry forests and savannah woodlands.

Description
Cashew apples are oblong-shaped and brightly coloured, with varying shades of yellow, orange, and red. The flavour is delicate, sweet, and slightly acidic. Ripe fruits are super juicy and very aromatic. Tastes like a cross between a grapefruit and a mango.

Culinary Use
Cashew pulp is frozen, dried, sweetened, or juiced. Fresh cashew apples are astringent and not palatable unless sprinkled with salt. The high pectin content in cashew apples makes them suitable for making jams, jellies, chutneys and preserves. They can be cooked in curries or fermented into vinegar or citric acid. In South America the cashew apples are used to flavour drinks.

Nutritional value
High in vitamin C and fibre, carbohydrates, some sugars, and minerals like calcium, magnesium, phosphorus, riboflavin, and thiamine.

Interesting facts and folklore
In the mid sixteenth century the tree was taken to Goa, India by the Portuguese traders. Fruits are famously fermented and distilled by the monks into an alcoholic brandy known as feni. Likewise in Brazil, a fermented drink called "cajuína" is made from cashew apple juice.

Cecropia
Cecropia peltata

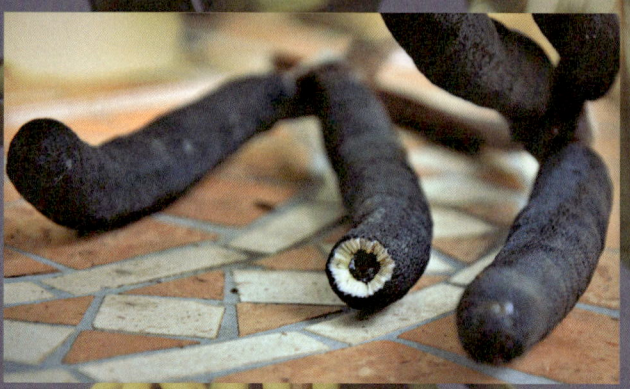

Other names
Trumpet tree, guarumo, snakewood, snake fingers, pumpwood, trumpet tree, snakewood, Congo pump, wild pawpaw, pop-a-gun ambay, yarumo, emajagua, yarumá, cedro macho, urraco.

Native habitat
The native range of this species is Mexico to northern Brazil, Jamaica to Barbados. Most species of Cecropia grow in lowland humid rainforests in Colombia and Ecuador, from sea level to 1,300m.

Description
Cecropia fruits are long and slender, growing in clusters at the end of short stems, like octopus arms or "snake fingers". They have a sweet, jelly-like flesh with a honey or fig flavour. There are several tiny seeds embedded in the long (7cm), drooping, greenish-grey, soft-fleshed fruiting stems.

Culinary Use
Fruit is eaten raw from the pods when ripe. Cecropia has a sweet, jelly-like flesh. They can be dried, or mostly they are eaten as a snack. The flesh from the fruits is used to make marmalade or jam, or as a flavouring for smoothies.

Nutritional value
The fruit and leaves are good sources of magnesium, potassium, iron and manganese.

Interesting facts and folklore
The astringent sap from the tree is applied externally to treat snake bites, scorpion stings, ulcers, warts and eczema. Aztecs sometimes make blowpipes and flutes from the hollow stems. Cecropia has a symbiotic relationship with the biting Aztec ants who protect the tree from herbivores.

Ceylon gooseberry
Dovyalis hebecarpa

Other names
Sri Lanka gooseberry, ketembilla, kitambilla, aberia, Puerto Rican cranberries, and tropical apricots.

Native habitat
It is native to Sri Lanka and southern India. It grows in the wet/dry tropics at sea level to 1200 metres. It grows well in a range of soils, including limestone.

Description
Fruits are small berries (2.5cm), pale green to orange when immature, ripening to a dark purple. They are sweetest when slightly wrinkled. They are seldom eaten fresh out of the hand, mainly due to the small fine hairs on the skins, but also due to their bitterness and strong acidity. They taste similar to an astringent apricot.

Culinary Use
Seldom eaten fresh due to their astringent taste. They are usually cooked into jams and jellies. They are commonly mixed with papaya to make jam and sauces. They can be pureed, used as a salad dressing, chutney, dipping sauce, wine, drinks, and barbeque sauce.

Nutritional value
Like most dark purple skinned fruits they are high in antioxidants and polyphenols. High in vitamin C.

Interesting facts and folklore
Anthocyanin pigments have been used in folk medicine to treat diarrhoea, infections, boost vision, inhibit tumours and cancers. Trees are often used as a boundary hedge due to its thorns.

Cherimoya
Annona cherimola

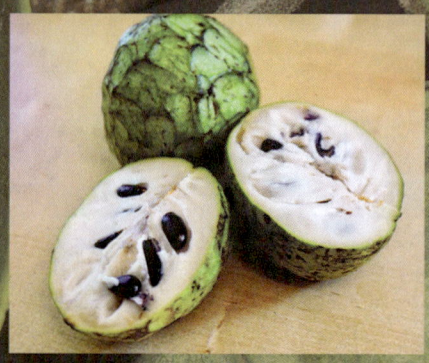

Other names
Cherimolier, custard apple, chirimoya, chirimuya.

Native habitat
Native to the highland valleys of the Andes Mountains of Ecuador and Peru. They are found wild in the Loja region of Ecuador, bordering Peru, in the low rising tropical forests of Central Andean Mountains.

Description
The white flesh of cherimoya is soft and sweet and has the flavour of mango, pawpaw, bananas and coconut. The large, oval or heart shaped, pale green fruits are smooth or have round protrusions, with a skin that gives the appearance of having overlapping scales. The flesh is white and pulpy, fragrant, with a strong, sweet acid flavour. A few black, bean-size seeds are embedded in the pulp.

Culinary Use
They're really delicious when served icy-cold from the freezer and eaten like ice-cream. Just chill it and spoon it out from the skin. Toss fresh cherimoya pulp in salads. Puree it for smoothies and sorbets, and to freeze for future use. Do not eat the seeds as they are poisonous so remove them before you put any fruit in the blender. Refrigerated fruit will last for three to five days.

Nutritional value
Cherimoyas are rich in vitamin C and B6, high in fibre, a very good source of carbohydrates, riboflavin, folate, thiamine, magnesium, vitamin E, zinc, manganese, phosphorus, and niacin.

Interesting facts and folklore
According to writer Mark Twain the cherimoya is *"the most delicious fruit known to men".* The name originates from the Quechua word chirimuya, which means "cold seeds".

Chinese jujube
Zizyphus jujuba

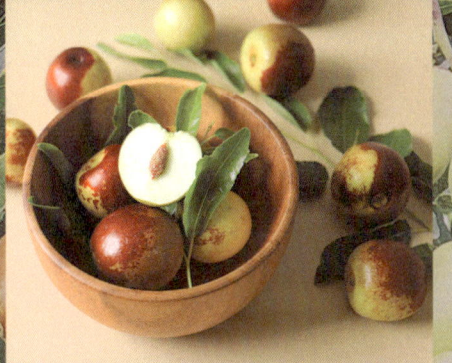

Other names
Chinese date, common jujube, red date, dounce, chinee apple, coolie plum, crabapple, Indian jujube, Indian cherry, Indian plum, masau, Taiwan apple.

Native habitat
Chinese jujubes are native from southwest Asia between Lebanon and central China.. They grow naturally on dry, gravelly or stony slopes of hills and mountains. They require hot summers and good rainfall for abundant fruiting.

Description
Jujubes are small, oval to round, sweet, crisp and reddish to golden brown. Fruits can be eaten fresh or if left to dry on the tree they can be eaten like dates, when they will be very sweet with an apple flavour. Immature fruit is a smooth green. When ripe, they're dark red or purple and appear slightly wrinkled like a small date. There is a single hard kernel like an olive pit.

Culinary Use
Fruits are juiced, pureed, and made into jam and chutney. They are also preserved in syrup and dried. They can be eaten fresh, candied, dried and processed into wine.

Nutritional value
Chinese jujubes are particularly rich in vitamin C, low in calories and high in fibre. They are a great source of minerals, including potassium, zinc, and phosphorus.

Interesting facts and folklore
Jujube fruits have been used for centuries in alternative medicine to treat insomnia and anxiety. They were cultivated in southern Asia by 9000 BC.

Coco plum
Chrysobalanus icaco

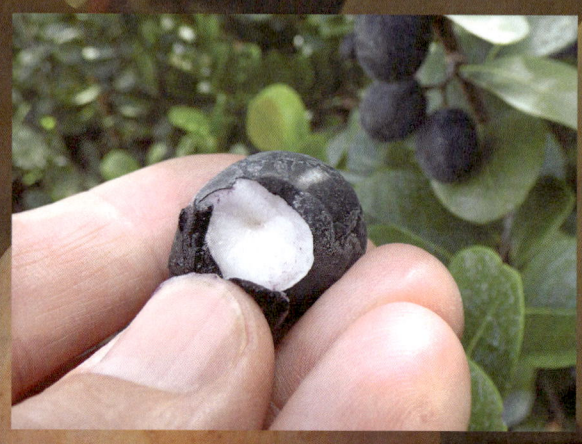

Other names
Icaco, paradise plum, abajeru, icaco, cacáo de praia (in Portuguese), golden plum, cocolmeca, pigeon plum, sea grape , yema, spicewood.

Native habitat
The cocoplum is a low shrub or small, bushy tree found near the beach and inland throughout tropical Africa, Americas, Caribbean, southern Florida and the Bahamas.

Description
There are 2 types, the coastal form being round (2.5-5 cm), thin skinned, pale-yellow with a rose blush or dark-purple in colour, while that of the inland form is oval (2.5 cm) and dark-purple. The edible fruit is juicy, sweet, and almost tasteless or insipid to mildly sweet flavour and a single stone. Purple or red-skinned fruits have a better flavour to white forms.

Culinary Use
Fruits are eaten raw or cooked. Better types have a fairly sweet, white, spongy flesh and are stewed in sugar, dried just like prunes or made into jellies and jams.

Nutritional value
Coco plums have vitamin C, calcium, iron, and phosphorus.

Interesting facts and folklore
The seeds are so rich in oil that they can be strung on sticks and burnt like a candle. The inland varieties have a pink 'Red Tip' or green 'Green Tip' blush on its new growth. The coastal type is used to stabilise sand dunes due to its creeping nature.

Cocona
Solanum sessiliflorum

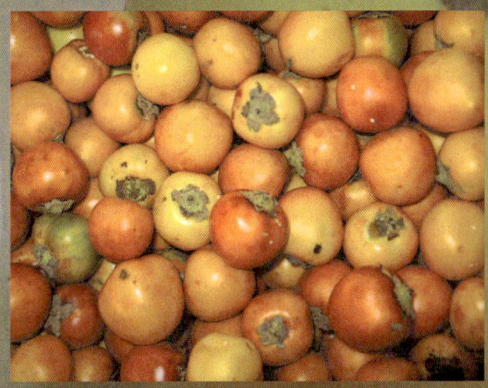

Other names
Orinoco apple, peach tomato, cubiu, tomate chauve souris (translates to "bat tomato") topiro.

Native habitat
Cocona is native to Brazil, Bolivia, Peru, and north through Central America to Mexico. It's native home is in the upper north western Amazon region in subtropical to tropical climates up to 1500 metres in elevation.

Description
The fruit of cocona is a red, orange or yellow edible berry. It has a fruity, acidic flavour, a pleasant taste of tomato with lemon. Cocona flesh ranges in colour from pale yellow to cream and is firm, dense, and aromatic, encasing an aqueous, jelly-like pulp with many tiny, flat, and oval seeds.

Culinary Use
Fruits can be eaten fresh out of hand but more usually peeled and used whole for making jams, jellies, preserves, pies, sauces. Juice from the pulp is mixed with ice and sugar to make refreshing drinks. Cocona fruit is also used as a vegetable in meat casseroles, with fish, salads and soups.

Nutritional value
Cocona is a good source of iron, an excellent source of vitamins A and C, and contains smaller amounts of phosphorus and calcium.

Interesting facts and folklore
Cocona has long been cultivated by the Amazon natives for its fruits. The juice of the boiled fruit has been taken to prevent vomiting, especially when it was caused by scorpion stings or spider bites.

Coconut
Cocos nucifera

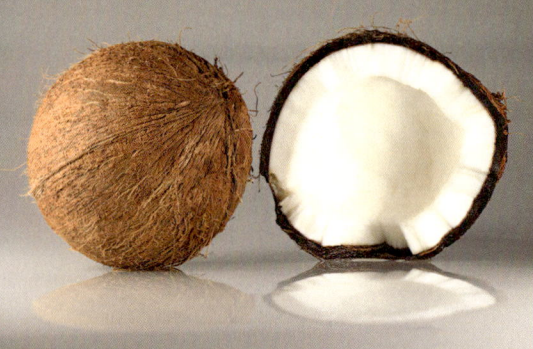

Other names
Copra, nariyal (in Hindi), narikel (in Bengali), kelapa (in Indonesian and Malay).

Native habitat
The coconut comes from the South Pacific, from the Philippines through Papua New Guinea and Indonesia to northern Australia.

Description
Coconuts have a glossy outer skin, yellow-green to yellow-brown in colour and a brown fibrous husk. The raw white meat inside a coconut is referred to as the kernel. It has a firm texture and delicious almost sweet flavour.

Culinary Use
The inner white meat as well as the coconut milk form a regular part of the diets of many people in the tropics. Dried coconut flesh is called copra, and the oil and milk derived from it are commonly used in cooking. The coconut sap can be made into drinks. It can also be fermented into palm wine or coconut vinegar. Coconut milk and cream are made from the raw, grated meat. Dried meat can be further processed and ground into flour.

Nutritional value
Coconut is high in carbohydrates, B vitamins, and manganese. It is rich in copper, iron, and selenium. Although coconut meat is high in fat, it also contains medium chain triglycerides that are metabolised differently than other types of fat. Coconut meat also provides protein.

Interesting facts and folklore
The palm fronds can be plaited into a wrap for the ketupat, a traditional Malay rice cake. Coconuts were a portable source of food and water, as well as providing building materials for outrigger boats.

Common guava
Psidium guava

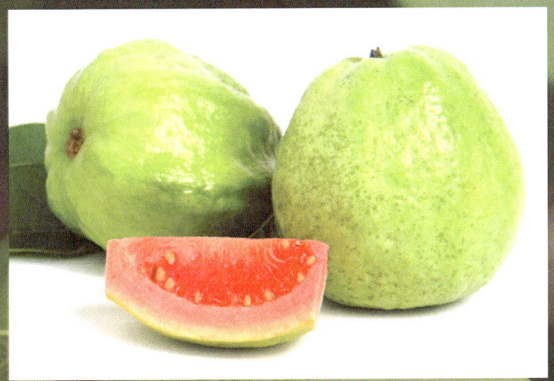

Other names
Guava, red guava, apple of the tropics, yellow guava, lemon guava, apple guava.

Native habitat
The common guava is native to the Caribbean, Central America and South America. It is found growing wild along forest margins, in rainforests, along the banks of watercourses, and in scrublands in higher rainfall areas.

Description
Guavas are generally green when immature, ripening to yellowish. Various cultivars have white, pink, or red flesh with a taste of a blend of pineapple, banana, papaya and lemon. They have a typical sharp fragrance, similar to lemon.

Culinary Use
Guava is eaten raw, cut into quarters or eaten like an apple, sometimes with a pinch of salt or pepper. They have a high level of pectin and are ideal for preserves, jellies and jams. They are often made into nectar or juice which is canned. The popular Mexican beverage agua fresca is commonly made with chopped guava, water, sugar and then blended.

Nutritional value
Guava fruits are amazingly rich in antioxidants, vitamin C and iron, and have good quantities of phosphorus and calcium. They are also a good source of fibre, potassium, and vitamin A.

Interesting facts and folklore
Guava wood is commonly used for the smoking of meat. The plant is used in many different shampoo products for its scent. It has oil glands that are harvested for essential oils.

Cuban mangosteen
Garcinia aristata

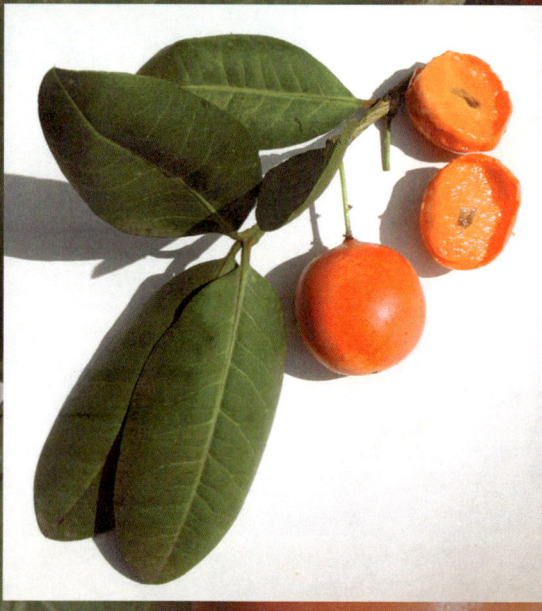

Other names
Palo de Cruz, manaju.

Native habitat
Native to Cuba, Hispaniola and Puerto Rico.

Description
Small orange-yellow fruits with a soft, sweet whitish or orange yellowish flesh. There are 1 or 2 large seeds.

Culinary Use
Flavour is very good, sweet with citrus tones and is edible fresh or in desserts and beverages.

Nutritional value
Rich in essential nutrients, including Vitamin C, Vitamin B9 (folate), Vitamin B1 (thiamine), Vitamin B2 (riboflavin), Manganese, Copper, and Magnesium.

Interesting facts and folklore
Xanthones show potential anti-inflammatory, anticancer, anti-aging, and antidiabetic effects.

Dabai
Canarium odontophyllum

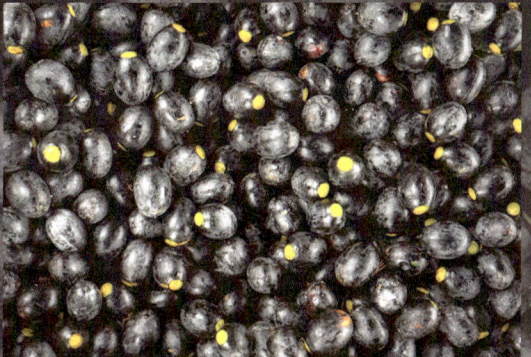

Other names
Kembayau, Sarawakian olive, buah dabai, sibu olive, or-kana (black olive in Hokkien).

Native habitat
Dabai is native to the tropical regions of Sarawak and Brunei. Its habitat includes the Rajang River in Sarawak, along hillsides, in fertile soils as a canopy tree in tropical lowland forests to an altitude of 700 metres in constant humidity.

Description
Clusters of olive-like fruits are held above the dark green foliage. Immature fruits are a startling white turning blue-black when ripe. They are oblong, 3.5-4 cm long, with a thin, edible skin. Flesh is yellow or white, and has a single, large 3-angled seed. It has a unique taste, and a thick, rich, oily texture like an avocado.

Culinary Use
Ripe dabai fruits are first soaked in hot water for ten minutes until they soften. They are good with some sugar for a quick snack, or eaten with salt or dipped in soy sauce as a savoury snack. Seeds are also edible and nutritious with a high oil content. Flavour has been likened to buttered carrots, olives, and brie cheese. Ripe, unsoftened fruits last for only 3 days at room temperature.

Nutritional value
Rich in unsaturated fats, protein and carbohydrates, Vitamin E, phosphorus, calcium, and magnesium.

Interesting facts and folklore
A great dish is called nasi goreng dabai, a dish of dabai and fried rice. There is an annual festival known as Pesta Dabai in honour of the fruit in Song, on the banks of the Katibas River in Sarawak.

Date
Phoenix dactylifera

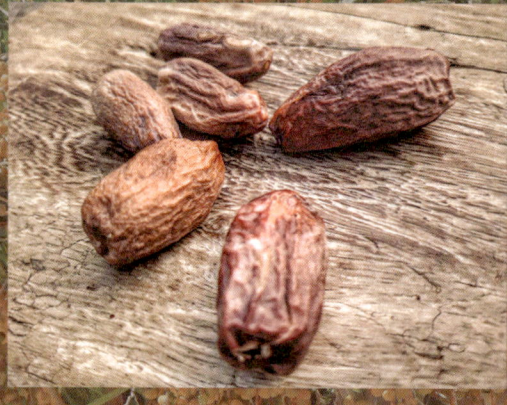

Other names
Date palm, edible date.

Native habitat
Dates are native to the Arabian Peninsula to southern Pakistan. Some say that they probably originated from the Fertile Crescent region straddling Egypt and Mesopotamia, while others state that they are native to the Persian Gulf area.

Description
Date fruits are oval (3-7cm long) and depending upon variety range from dark brown to bright red or yellow. They grow in clusters of large, edible sweet fruits and have a thick layer of fruit pulp. Fruits are green when unripe, then change to a yellow, golden brown, red, or black when they ripen. It is a one-seeded fruit.

Culinary Use
Dates are used to make vinegar, syrups and a strong liquor. They contain a large amount of sugar by mass when dried. Consequently they are very sweet and are enjoyed as desserts on their own or within sweets. Dates are eaten fresh or dried out-of-hand, or they may be pitted and stuffed with fillings such as walnuts.

Nutritional value
Dates are a rich source of potassium. They are a moderate source of pantothenic acid, vitamin B6, magnesium and manganese. They contain carbohydrates, of which consist mostly of sugars and some dietary fibre.

Interesting facts and folklore
Upwards of 1,000 dates may appear on a single bunch weighing 8 kg or more. In Africa the leaves are used to make huts, mats, baskets and fans.

Downy rose cherry
Rhodomyrtus tomentosa

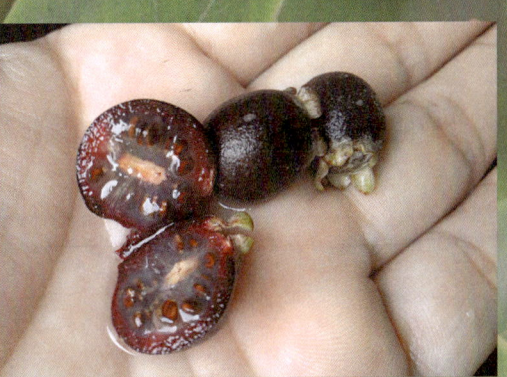

Other names
Rose myrtle, Ceylon hill gooseberry, downy myrtle, downy rose myrtle.

Native habitat
Trees are said to be native to southern and south eastern Asia from India east to southern China and the Philippines and south to Sulawesi and Malaysia. It is an important environmental weed because it forms large thickets that displace native flora and fauna. It grows in natural and regrowth forests, wetlands, and bog margins from 0-2400m in elevation.

Description
The fruits are green when immature and ripen to a purplish-black colour. They are egg-shaped berries. Each fruit contains 40 or more seeds. Ripe fruits have a sweet taste reminiscent of blueberries, raspberries or grapes. They are aromatic.

Culinary Use
Select the darkest purple fruits for eating fresh as they are the sweetest. Ceylon hill cherries are usually eaten raw, or made into jellies and pies. Fruit are particularly good made into wine, tea and jam. In Vietnam the fresh fruits are canned with syrup for export.

Nutritional value
Fruit is considered very healthy with anthocyanins and antioxidants . They have high levels of total dietary fibre, potassium, calcium, manganese, iron, zinc and copper.

Interesting facts and folklore
The fruit has been used as a cure for dysentery and diarrhoea. The tar from the wood along with coconut shells can serve as a black dye and has been used to blacken teeth and eyebrows. In China cherries are used for the treatment of urinary tract infections.

Durian
Durio zibethinus

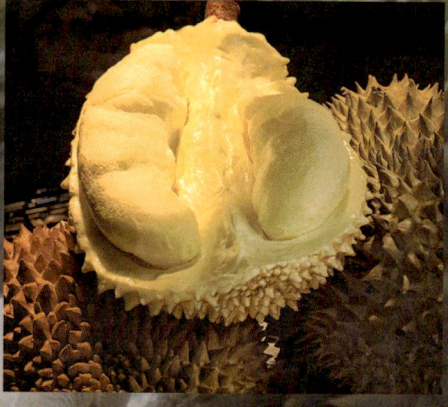

Other names:
King of fruits, 'Skunk of the orchard', 'civet fruit', doerian, dulian, duren, durian kampong.

Native habitat:
Durio sp. are native to Borneo and Sumatra. They are a tropical species and prefer humid lowland climes with regular rainfall throughout the year.

Description:
The durian fruit is a large, round to oval spiky fruit with a tough outside shell and creamy pale yellow flesh divided into segments. The yellowish-green rind is thick, tough and covered with stout, sharply pointed spines. It has a very unique flavour that combines sweet, savoury and is accompanied by a strong aroma. Each fruit has several large brown seeds.

Culinary Use:
Durians are usually eaten fresh by themselves or with sticky glutinous rice steamed in coconut milk or sugar. Tempoyak is a good way of using lower quality durian. It is made by frying the flesh until it turns brown and serving it as a side dish with a meal. Freshly fallen fruit has a shelf life of up to 8 days. Durian ice cream is a treat.

Nutritional value:
Durian is rich in carbohydrates, healthy fats, fibre, vitamins C and B, and essential minerals potassium, magnesium, and copper.

Interesting facts and folklore
The durian is adored by many people in its native homeland, some are willing to walk miles to roadside stalls in order to obtain these freshly fallen delights.

Gamboge
Garcinia xanthochymus

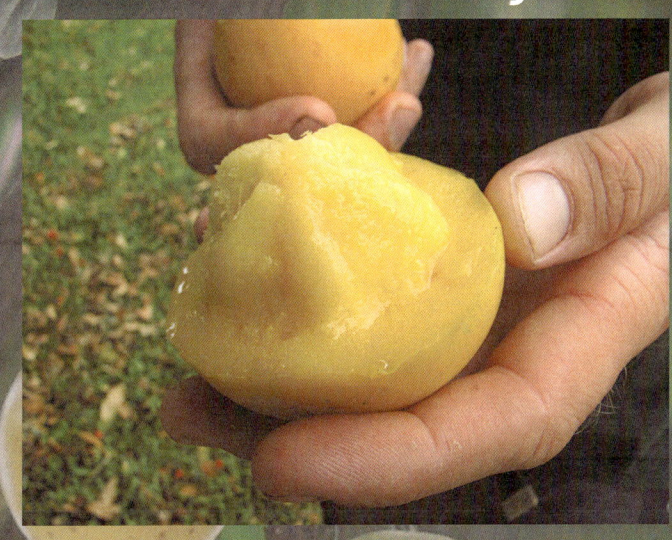

Other names
False mangosteen, yellow mangosteen, Himalayan garcinia, sour mangosteen.

Native habitat
Gamboge is native to Bangladesh, Bhutan, Cambodia, India, Laos, Myanmar, Nepal, Thailand, and Vietnam. It grows wild in dense, humid forests in the tropics at altitudes of 600 - 1,000 metres above sea level.

Description
Gamboge fruit are bright yellow-orange, roundish, and 5 - 9 cm in diameter. The fleshy fruit contains around 5 seeds that are surrounded by an edible yellow pulp. The thin skinned fruit is rather sour.

Culinary Use
Gamboge has a pleasant acid taste, usually eaten as a breakfast fruit. They are used in sherbets, jams, curries and vinegar or as a flavouring agent.

Nutritional value
Gamboge is rich in vitamin C with antioxidant properties due to the presence of xanthone. It has dietary fibre, vitamin A, iron, and calcium.

Interesting facts and folklore
Gamboge contains a resin, a yellow pigment extracted from the tree, which has been used as a paint ingredient and to dye the yellow silken robes of Buddhists monks.

Giant granadilla
Passiflora quadrangularis

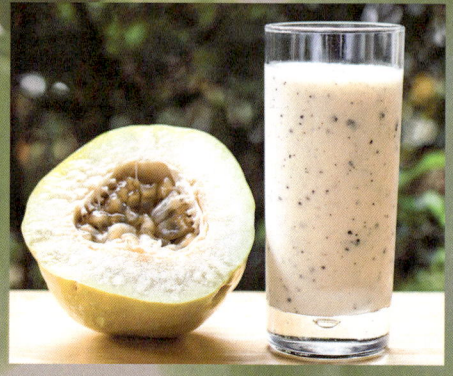

Other names
Giant passionfruit, badia, sweet granadilla, curuba, tumbo.

Native habitat
Native range of habitat is likely in tropical America from Colombia to Brazil.

Description
They are large yellow, melon-shaped or oval fruits or berries (10-30cm long), with purple pulp. Fruit skin is greenish white to pale yellow and thin. The flesh is white or pink and the cavity contains juice and yellowish sweet-acidic pulp enclosing flat, oval, brown seeds. Fruits turn yellow when fully ripe. Pulp doesn't have the flavour of the common passionfruit.

Culinary Use
The fruit juice of the giant granadilla is used as a drink, cooked as a vegetable curry, and the seeds eaten as a snack. The flesh of green, unripe fruit can be cooked like squash as a vegetable substitute. The moist yellowish pulp can be eaten fresh or used in drinks, fruit salad or desserts. Scoop out the sweet and aromatic pulp with a spoon. The fruit flesh (with inner skin removed) can be diced and added to fruit salads.

Nutritional value
The pulp contains calcium, phosphorus, iron, vitamin A and C, and niacin.

Interesting facts and folklore
The giant granadilla is the biggest fruit of the *Passiflora* genus. The rind is used to treat headaches, asthma, diarrhoea, dysentery, and insomnia. Seeds are a sedative and in large doses a narcotic. The giant granadilla is not to be confused with its relative the sweet granadilla (*Passiflora ligularis*) which is native in a wide belt from northern Argentina to Central America.

Green sapote
Pouteria viridis

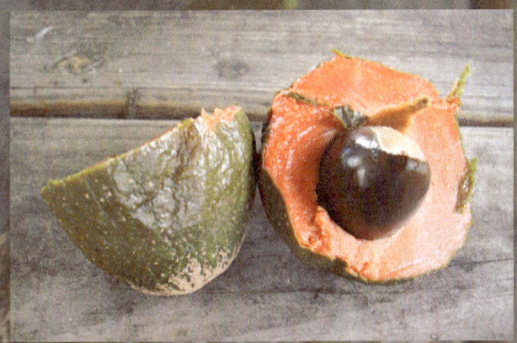

Other names
Zapotilla calenturiento, zapote amarillo, zapote mico, zapote real, chulul, red faisan, white faisan, zapote verde (green sapote).

Native habitat
Native to the frost free highland regions of Central America. Its native habitat includes areas in southern Mexico, Guatemala, and El Salvador. It loves the well drained volcanic soils in the mountainous regions of Central America. Trees grow in the equatorial regions but they are adapted to cooler subtropical conditions up to altitudes of 2100m.

Description
The round, dark brownish-green fruit turns to a red, orange or gold when ripe. Fruit softens when ripe and the thick orange fine textured flesh melts in your mouth. Green sapote has a better flavour and finer texture to its close relative the mamey sapote. The pulp is sweet and a bit juicy and contains up to 1 to 2 dark brown, shiny, edible seeds.

Culinary Use
Green sapote are delicious eaten fresh out of hand, in milkshakes, or served with ice cream. The pulp is also used in making preserves and dessert dishes.

Nutritional value
Green sapotes are a good source of vitamin A and C and are high in carbohydrates. They also contain calcium, iron, potassium, and magnesium.

Interesting facts and folklore
The latex of the tree can be made into chewing gum and has been applied to the skin to treat warts and fungal infections. The seeds are edible and commonly roasted. The bark has anti-termite properties.

Guavaberry
Myrciaria florabunda

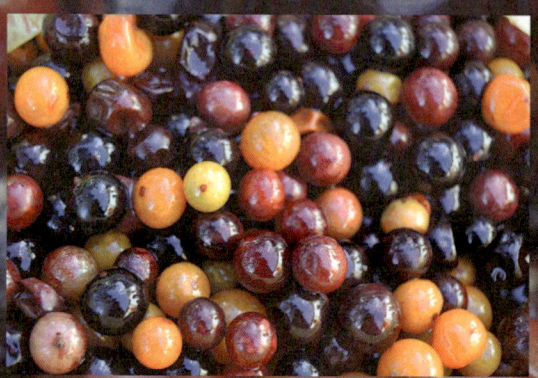

Other names
Rumberry, cambuizeiro, mirto (in Puerto Rico), guaveberry (in St. Martin and St. Eustatius), guayabillo (in Guatemala), bay berry.

Native habitat
Native to Central and South America (through Northern Brazil), and the Caribbean. It grows in dry or moist coastal woodlands up to 300 metres above sea level.

Description
Guavaberry fruits (1cm) are green when immature and ripen to yellow-orange, deep red, or purple-black. They are half the size of a cherry and have a sweet to acid taste. The translucent, yellow-orange flesh surrounds a single, roundish seed.

Culinary Use
Unripe fruits are very sour but ripen to sweet-acid when ripe and are made into jellies, jams, fruit drinks, and baked in pies and cakes. Their main use is a flavouring agent in a local alcoholic drink known as guavaberry liqueur. It is a dark red liqueur with a woody, bitter-sweet flavour used in Caribbean cocktails.

Nutritional value
Guavaberries have large amounts of vitamin C, approximately 30 times higher than oranges. They also have fibre, vitamin B and iron, niacin, phosphorus, riboflavin and thiamin.

Interesting facts and folklore
Guavaberry is the legendary folk rum of St Maarten. It was made hundreds of years ago in people's homes out of fine oak aged rum, cane sugar and guavaberries picked by hand to assure ripeness. The fruit grew wild in the hills on the island.

Herbert river cherry
Antidesma dallachyanum

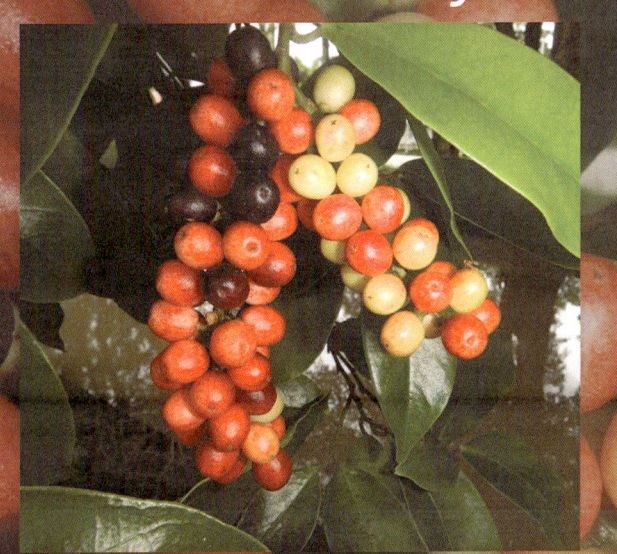

Other names
Current tree, wild cherry.

Native habitat
Herbert river cherry is native to northern Australia.

Description
Fruits are round to oval up to 2cm in diameter. The red immature fruits turn black when ripe and are sweet with pleasant acidity. One of the best Antidesma species in terms of fruit quality. Bears hundreds of small reddish fruits. Similar to its close relative the bignay but with more flesh. Aroma similar to apples.

Culinary Use
They can be eaten fresh or used for making juices and jams. The juice is very dark-red, nearly black. Add some pectin to it to make a deep-red jelly. A fruit vinegar is made from the cherries.

Nutritional value
Berries are high in vitamin C, flavonoids and phenolic acids making them a natural antioxidant. Also high in fibre and manganese.

Interesting facts and folklore
It is rich in antioxidants and has traditionally been used for digestion, skin and inflammation issues.

Ilama
Annona macrophyllata

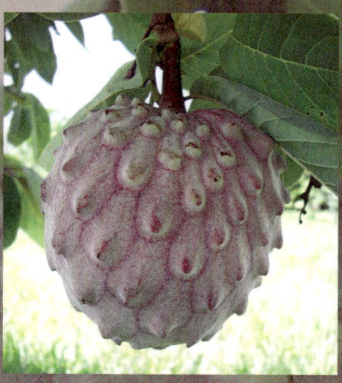

Other names
Soncoya, sincuya, ilamatzapotil, red ilama, izlama, papausa.

Native habitat
Ilama comes from the mountains and foothills of south western Mexico, Guatemala, and El Salvador. The trees are tropical and don't like near zero temperatures. It is commonly described as being the cherimoya of the lowlands.

Description
The oval-shaped fruit has a thick, rough, surface with scale-like protuberances, typical of the *Annona* family. Skin colour varies from pale green to purple and is coated with a velvety greyish bloom. The flesh may be white (sweet) or reddish-pink (tart). The flesh is soft, aromatic and creamy with a custardy texture. There are numerous brown-black, smooth inedible seeds.

Culinary Use
Chill fruits, halve them and scoop the flesh out of the rind. Serve them with cream and sugar to intensify the flavour, or with a drop of lime juice for a tart taste. Fruits are best left on the tree until they begin to crack open for best flavour and sweetness.

Nutritional value
Ilama is rich in vitamin C, dietary fibre, calcium and phosphorus. High in amino acids like lysine, methionine, threonine and tryptophan.

Interesting facts and folklore
The name ilama is derived from the Nahuatl *ilamatzapotl*, which translates as zapote de las viejas, "old woman's sapote". Scratch the bark of a branch and the colour will hint at the colour of the flesh. If it's green the flesh is white, red and the flesh will be pink.

Imbe
Garcinia livingstonei

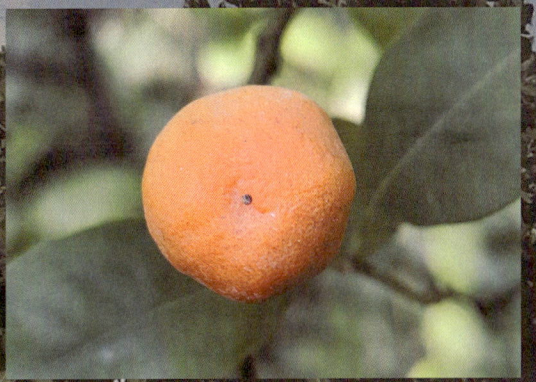

Other names
African mangosteen, wild African plum, African mangosteen, lowveld mangosteen, Livingstone's garcinia.

Native habitat
Native to a broad region of tropical Africa from Cote d'Ivoire east to Somalia, and south to South Africa. Grows in drier areas, in riverine woodland or on rocky outcrops away from water, river banks in dry hilly areas from sea level to 1,900 metres.

Description
Fruit is small, thick skinned and plum-like, bright orange when fully ripe. A thin layer of juicy, acid-sweet pulp surrounds the seed similar to achacha. Fruit is good if you leave it long enough on the tree. Simply picking after it turns yellow is not good enough as they need to be more orange coloured. They have a pleasant, acidic, sweet flavour. Usually one seeded, occasionally two. Seeds are creamy brown.

Culinary Use
The juicy fruit pulp is acid-sweet, pleasant tasting and refreshing but with an aftertaste. They are eaten raw or cooked with porridge. You can crush them like grapes to create a drink. If you simply wash the fruit, cut them in half, scoop out the pulp and add it to a fruit salad or smoothie. Simply cook the fruit down with some sugar and water and make jam.

Nutritional value
Imbe fruit is rich in antioxidants, such as vitamin C, carotenoids, and polyphenols.

Interesting facts and folklore
An infusion made from roots has been used to treat stomach pains during pregnancy and after giving birth.

Indian gooseberry
Phyllanthus emblica

Other names
Emblic myrobalan, myrobalan, Malacca tree, amla (from the Sanskrit word amalaki, meaning "sour").

Native habitat
Indian gooseberry is native to India. It is found growing naturally along hill slopes, on exposed slopes and in dry deciduous forests from 800-1500m.

Description
Indian gooseberry fruits are light green, smooth, round, and about the size of a golf ball with a small hexagonal pit with 6 seeds. They have a sour, bitter, and astringent taste with some fibre. The skin is almost translucent with six faint striations making fruits appear segmented. They have tough, thin skins and a crisp and juicy pulp.

Culinary Use
Indian gooseberries can be eaten raw with salt or cooked. Fruit is often pickled with salt, oil, and spices. In northern India it is usually preserved in sugar and is called amla murabba and served with flatbreads. It has a high pectin content and is great for jam making.

Nutritional value
The fruit is rich in vitamin C, approximately 20 times more than oranges. They have antioxidants, phenols, flavonoids and tannins. It has calcium, phosphorus, iron, carotene and vitamin B complex.

Interesting facts and folklore
Indian gooseberry extract amla oil is commonly used in Thailand to promote hair growth. An oil is extracted from the dry berries that have been soaked in coconut oil. It was one of the first natural hair conditioners. It is said in India that after eating gooseberries a glass of water tastes sweet.

Inga
Inga edulis

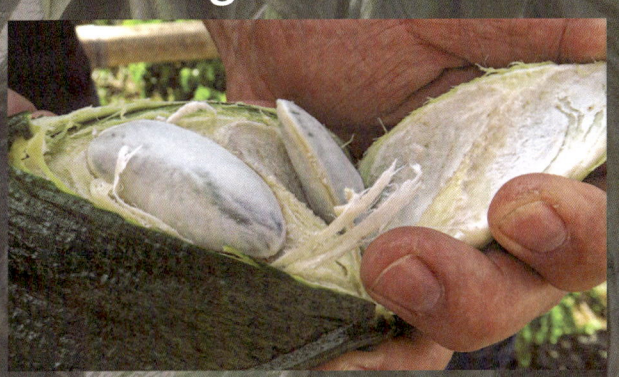

Other names
Ice-cream-bean, guama, guaba, guaba de bejuco or paterna, joaquiniquil, cuaniquil, monkey tamarind, monkey tail, pacay, buah salji (Indonesian for snow fruit).

Native habitat
The natural distribution of Inga edulis spreads from Central to South America and ranges from subtropical dry to tropical wet conditions. It can be found at elevations from sea level up to 2200m.

Description
Inga beans pods vary in length (50-100cm) with curved ends and raised ridges extending down the full velvety length. Surrounding the black seeds is a thick, creamy white, juicy sweet pulp that tastes very much like vanilla ice-cream. It's the fluffy white seed coating that everyone loves to suck off each seed. Seeds are toxic raw, but commonly eaten cooked with a nut-like or chickpea flavour. Fruit keeps for only 3-4 days in the fruit bowl but up to 3 weeks in the refrigerator.

Culinary Use
The white pulp is commonly consumed raw as a sweet snack. In Colombia the flesh is also used to prepare an alcoholic beverage called cachiri. It is used in salads especially with avocado, smoothies, chocolates, candies, juices, and syrups. Pulp is not usually cooked.

Nutritional value
Inga beans are a good source of fibre, calcium, phosphorous, iron, vitamin C and B.

Interesting facts and folklore
Inga species have a symbiotic relationship with ants which farm the nectar. In exchange the ants will patrol over the Inga plant to protect it against herbivores. Seed remnants have been found in tombs dating back to 1000 BCE.

Jaboticaba
Myrciaria cauliflora

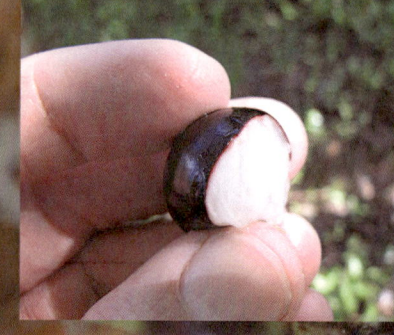

Other names
Brazilian grape tree, jabuticaba, yvapurŭ, iba-puru, guapuru, yabuticaba de campinas.

Native habitat
Jaboticaba is native to the hilly region around Rio de Janeiro and Minas Gerais, Brazil, also around Santa Cruz, Bolivia, Asunción, Paraguay, and northeastern Argentina. It grows wild from sea level to 1000 metres in Brazil.

Description
Purple, grape-like fruits (3-4cm) grow straight on the trunk and main branches after the tiny white flowers are pollinated. The smooth, tough skin is glossy, maroon-purple, almost black. Flesh is gelatinous, juicy, translucent, and rose-tinted and clings firmly to the seeds. Jaboticabas are subacid to sweet, with a grape-like flavour. There are 1-4 small seeds.

Culinary Use
If you squeeze the fruit between your thumb and forefinger, it causes the skin to burst and the pulp to slide out for eating fresh out of the hand. Ripe fruits are highly nutritious and are mostly eaten as fresh fruit but are also processed to make juice, liquor, dry sweet wine, vinegar, sherbets, jam, jelly, tarts and marmalade (add pectin). Fruits ferment after 3 or 4 days so shelf life is short.

Nutritional value
Jaboticaba is high in carbohydrates, fibre, vitamins C, flavonoids and minerals calcium, potassium, and magnesium. The skin is rich in antioxidants, specifically anthocyanins and tannins.

Interesting facts and folklore
Traditionally, the sun-dried skins have been used as a treatment for diarrhoea, asthma and chronic inflammation of the tonsils. Jaboticaba has become popular as a bonsai plant in Taiwan.

Jackfruit
Artocarpus heterophyllus

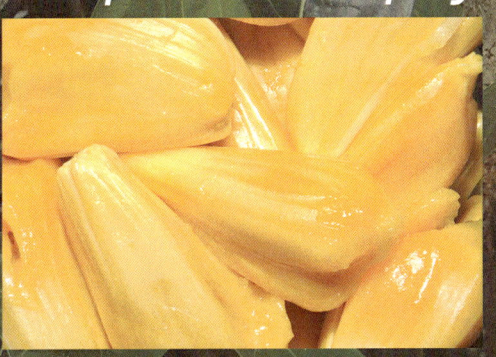

Other names
Jakfruit, jak, jaca, nangka, khanun, khnor, maki mi, may mi, mit, kathal.

Native habitat
Jackfruit are evergreen, latex-producing trees native to the rainforests of the western Ghats (mountains) of India. The tree thrives in hot, humid environments with high rainfall and cannot tolerate dry or cold conditions. Grows well in lowland rainforests and moist, well-drained soils.

Description
Jackfruit are large to very large fruits, oblong in shape, ranging from 10-60 cm long and 25-75 cm in diameter. The thick rind is covered in small spikes. Fruits are green when unripe, turning brownish-yellow when ripe. Flesh is yellow-orange in colour. There are numerous seeds, 100 to 500 per fruit depending upon size.

Culinary Use
Jackfruit is eaten fresh, dried, or preserved in syrup. It's commonly served in salads. The fleshy segments enclosing the seeds is the choicest part of the fruit, however the stringy "rags" in between are also tasty. The seeds can be boiled or roasted. Unripe fruit is used as a vegetable in soups or baked/fried in dishes.

Nutritional Value
Jackfruit is a source of fibre, protein and vitamin B and contains potassium, iron and calcium. The deep yellow-orange flesh is rich in beta carotene.

Interesting facts and folklore
Jackfruit has been cultivated in India 3000 to 6000 years ago and has played a significant role in their agriculture for centuries. In Kerala, India, an ornate wooden plank called *avani palaka*, made of Jackfruit wood, is used as the priest's seat during Hindu ceremonies.

Jelly palm
Butia capitata

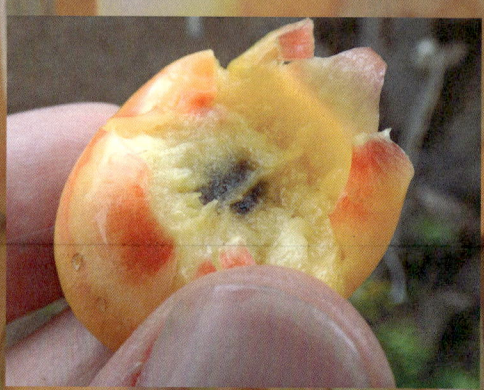

Other names
Pindo palm, yatay palm, butia palm, wine palm.

Native habitat
Jelly palm is native to subtropical regions of South America, in the southeastern parts of Brazil, Uruguay, and northern Argentina. It grows wild usually together in large numbers in grasslands, savannas, and along deciduous forest margins.

Description
Jelly palm fruit is green prior to ripening, then turns gold, sometimes having a yellowish or reddish tinge when ripe. It is about the size of a large cherry and has a soft, tasty flesh surrounding a hard seed that looks like a small coconut. Peel the flesh away and eat it fresh, prepare a puree, or use it in a jelly. The taste is delicious with apple and tropical flavours. They are eaten fresh but they are mostly preserved due to their stringy, fibrous flesh. They keep well in the refrigerator for 7 days.

Culinary Use
The fruit can be eaten fresh but is also used to make jelly and wine, hence the name jelly or wine palm.

Nutritional value
The pulp is a good source of beta-carotene and provitamin A . A glass of juice containing jelly palm pulp can provide almost half of the daily vitamin A requirements for children.

Interesting facts and folklore
The *Butia capitata* is named the wine and jelly palm because its seeds have fruit around them that are edible and taste like wine and jelly.

Kaffir plum
Harpephyllum caffrum

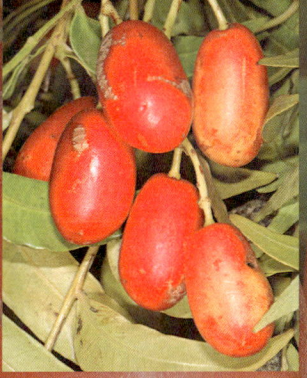

Other names
Marula plum, African marula, elephant tree, jelly plum, marriage tree, maroela (in Afrikaans), umganu (in Zulu), wild plum, South African plum.

Native habitat
Native to eastern parts of Southern Africa, from the Cape, through Mozambique and Zimbabwe.

Description
These small (2-3cm) oval-shaped, plum-like fruits grow in bunches resembling grapes. They are smooth, glossy and green when immature and ripen to a deep red colour. Kaffir plums have juicy orange flesh with a single large seed. Not much flesh but it is easily separated from the seed. The flesh is pleasantly tart or sour and is very aromatic. Taste is similar to mango or passionfruit.

Culinary Use
Kaffir plums are commonly used to make jams, jellies and preserves like chutney. The tardiness of the fresh fruit is used in soft drinks. Juice is commonly fermented into a rose wine.

Nutritional value
High in fibre, and a good source of vitamin C and A, potassium and antioxidants.

Interesting facts and folklore
The bark burnt to a powder has been used as a topical agent against acne, skin and eczema. Smoke from burning roots has been used by spiritualists to ward off demons. The wood is used for carving and furniture. Wild animals like monkeys, baboons, bats and bushbabies picnic on these tart fruits.

Karonda
Carissa carandas

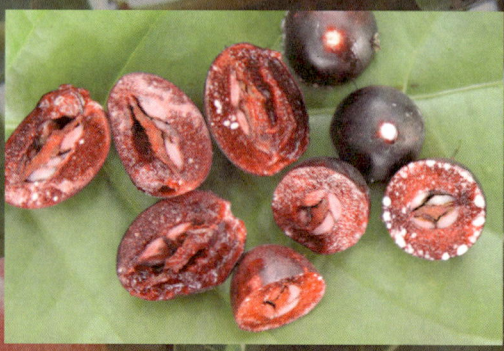

Other names
Bengal currant, Christ's thorn, carandas plum, karanda, and kanna, kerenda, karaunda, caramba, caranda, caraunda, perunkila, nam phrom, nam daeng.

Native habitat
Primarily found in India, particularly the Western Ghats and the Himalayan foothills. It's also found in the lowland rainforests of Sri Lanka, Pakistan, Nepal, Afghanistan, and Bangladesh.

Description
The small, round, berry-sized fruit changes from green or buff to a wrinkled, red or pink and finally dark purple colour when ripe. The velvety skin is slightly rough. Inside, the flesh is pale red or translucent with 3 to 5 seeds. They have a sweet to acid taste, reminiscent of mango, pineapple, and banana.

Culinary Use
In India, the mature fruit is harvested for pickles and chutneys. The fruit is also used as a substitute for cherries in cakes and other desserts, and it was processed into candied murabba, jams, jellies, and syrups by colonial British in India. It can be eaten raw or stewed with sugar. In Thailand it is pickled or made into jams, jellies and puddings.

Nutritional value
Carissa carandas is rich in iron, vitamin C, vitamins A, calcium and phosphorus.

Interesting facts and folklore
The fruit of the plant is utilised in Ayurvedic medicine for treating various ailments such as acidity, indigestion, wounds, skin diseases, urinary disorders, and diabetic ulcers. A sturdy shrub, it was used in the Great Hedge of India (1803-1879 A.D.) to prevent smuggling.

Kei apple
Dovyalis caffra

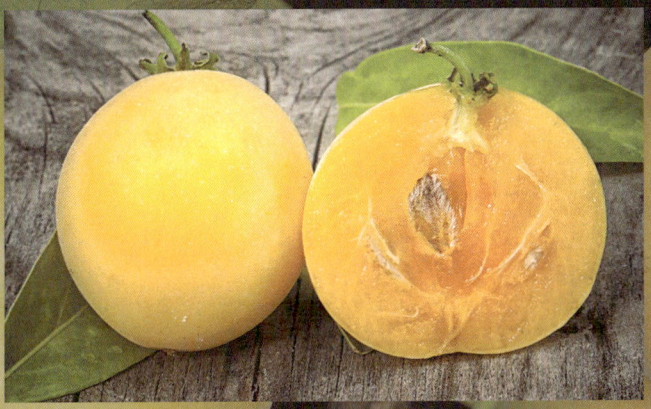

Other names
Umkokolo (Zulu), kayaba, kai apple, kau apple, wild apricot.

Native habitat
Native to the Kei River area of southwest Africa and can be found growing wild in Swaziland, Mozambique, and Zimbabwe.

Description
Fruits are small, round and plum sized. The skin is smooth, velvety, and semi-tough, ripening from green to orange and golden when mature. Underneath the surface, the golden flesh is soft, watery, and succulent, and with a sweet scent. Fruits contain 5 to 15 seeds. They are sweet to acid and taste very similar to an apricot but with a much higher juice content.

Culinary Use
Fruit is not often eaten out of hand and its primary use is as an ingredient in preserves and jellies. They are also used in desserts, or pickled. Kei apple slices can also be used in fruit or green salads or baked into cakes, puddings, tarts, and pies. They can be made into a tasty fruit leather.

Nutritional value
High in vitamin C (twice that of an orange), potassium, phosphorus, and fibre. They contain 7 out of the 9 essential amino acids. High in pectin.

Interesting facts and folklore
Kei apple is cultivated as an impenetrable hedge for protection when close planted. Dovyalis is a Greek word meaning spear and caffra comes from Kaffraria in the Eastern Cape. Baboons, monkeys and antelopes love the fruit.

Key lime
Citrus aurantiifolia

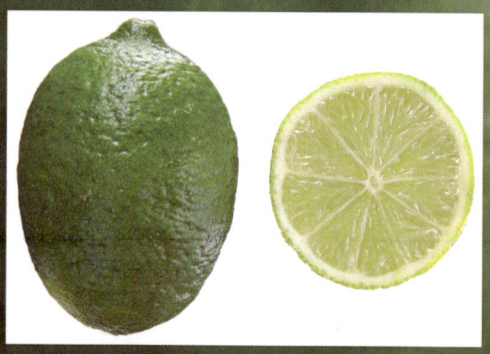

Other names
West Indian lime, bartender's lime, Mexican lime (Limón Mexicano), dayap (Filipino), manao (Thai), chanh (Vietnamese), limão galego (Portuguese), tilleul clé (French).

Native distribution
Key limes are native to Southeast Asia, Indo-Malay region. They then spread through the Middle East to North Africa, on to Sicily and Andalucia. Spanish explorers took them to the West Indies, including the Florida Keys.

Description
Key limes are small, round or oval-shaped citrus fruits. They have thin, smooth, and greenish-yellow skin that turns slightly yellow when fully ripe. The flesh is juicy and acidic, distinctly tart with a refreshing citrusy flavour. They are usually more aromatic, tangy, with more seeds compared to Persian limes. The Key lime is usually picked while it is still green, but it becomes yellow when ripe.

Culinary Use
Fruits are famous for Key lime pie, a dessert known for its sweet-tart flavour and creamy texture. Additionally, they are used in limeade, cocktails such as margaritas, marinades, salad dressings, and as a garnish for seafood dishes.

Nutritional value
Key limes are rich in essential nutrients like vitamin C, folate, potassium, zinc, iron, calcium, and phosphorus.

Interesting facts and folklore
The Key Lime Festival in Key West, Florida, has been an annual event since 2002, held over the Independence Day weekend. Key limes are made into black lime (Middle East condiment) by boiling them in brine.

Kiwifruit
Actinidia chinensis

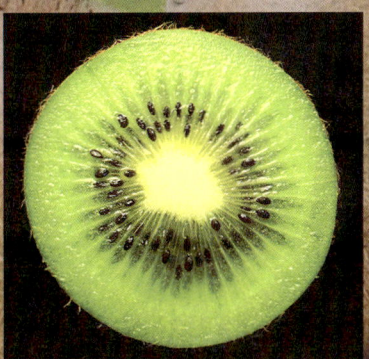

Other names
Chinese gooseberry, monkey peach, macaque pear, vine pear, sun peach, wood berry.

Native habitat
Kiwifruit is native to central and eastern China. This species thrives in subtropical mountainous regions at elevations from 200 to 2,600m, preferring habitats like mountain forests, thickets, secondary forests, and tall grassy areas. It prefers a subtropical to temperate climate with warm, humid summers and mild winters with plenty of rainfall throughout the year.

Description
Kiwifruit is a small, oval-shaped fruit with smooth, brown to bronze-coloured skin and a beaky shaped tip. Inside, the flesh ranges from bright green to yellow, with rows of tiny black, edible seeds arranged in a starburst pattern. It has a sweet to tart flavour with some acidity, and it ripens to a soft texture.

Culinary Use
It is great in salads, yoghurt parfaits, or smoothies. Use chopped or pureed in desserts like cakes, muffins, pies. Pairs well with other fruits like bananas, berries and mangoes and adds a unique twist to salads with cheese, chicken, or seafood. Ripe fruit can be refrigerated for up to 10 days.

Nutritional value
It's packed with vitamin C, exceeding even lemons in content and offering double the vitamin C of oranges. It's high in potassium compared to bananas. Rich in fibre, it also provides vitamin A, vitamin E, calcium, and iron.

Interesting facts and folklore
The fruit is often associated with prosperity, good fortune, and abundance due to its golden colour and sweetness.

Kwai muk
Artocarpus hypargyaeus

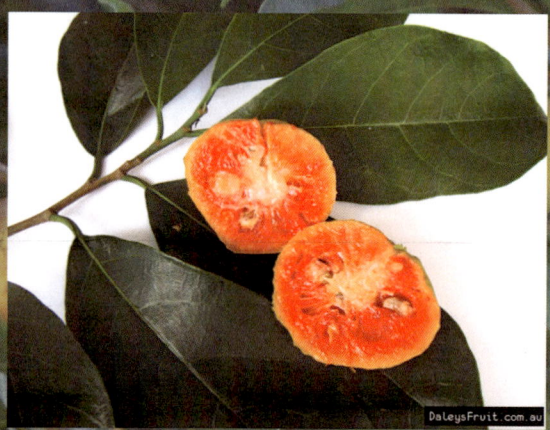

Other names
Green jackfruit, silver-back artocarpus, sweet artocarpus, ai gui mu, pai Klein mu.

Native habitat
The kwai muk is from China, where its native range includes southern Kwangtung Province, Hainan Island and Hong Kong. It grows best in well drained soils above 150 metres altitude in the tropics.

Description
Fruits are compact, plum sized and typically 1-2 inches (2.5-5 cm) in diameter. They vary in shape from round, egg-shaped, or flattened. They are thin skinned, velvety, and brown when unripe. They have a white latex sap until fully ripened. Ripe flesh is orange-red to red, soft, tender, and juicy. It has a nice tart or sweet-acidic flavour.

Culinary Use
The fruit is commonly eaten fresh, either on its own or as part of fruit salads. Kwai Muk is often used in desserts, smoothies, or milkshakes due to its sweet and creamy texture. It can be preserved by making jams or fruit preserves.

Nutritional value
It is a good source of vitamin C, provides minerals such as potassium, calcium and magnesium and is rich in dietary fibre and antioxidants.

Interesting facts and folklore
The stems, leaves and green fruits exude a white, sticky latex when they are cut or broken.

Langsat
Lansium domesticum

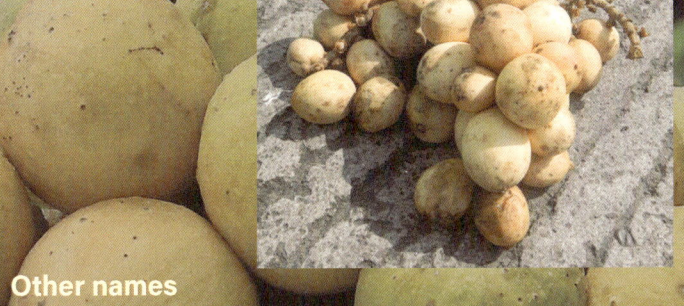

Other names
Lanzones, buah langsat, longkong, duku.

Native habitat
Native to western Malesia, it grows wild in the forests of southern Sumatra. It is very tropical, growing in the humid lowlands.

Description
The fruits can be elliptical, oval, or round. They are pale yellow or light brown when ripe, and form long drooping clusters. Ripe fruit develops a brown scurf on its thin skin. They usually have a sweet-tart flavour, slight acidity, similar to grapefruit and pomelo.

Culinary Use
It is eaten fresh, made into candies, preserved in syrup, and processed into wine. At room temperature, they can last for 3-4 days, and when stored in a refrigerator, they can keep for up to 7 days. Place freshly picked fruit in a cool spot in a fruit bowl and occasionally moisten them to prevent drying out.

Nutritional value
Langsats have good amounts of fibre, vitamin C, thiamin, riboflavin, niacin and folates, calcium, phosphorus and iron.

Interesting facts and folklore
The resin from the tree is non-toxic and used against diarrhoea and intestinal pain. Dried skins have been used in the treatment of diarrhoea, malaria, and fever. The bark is poulticed on scorpion stings, dysentery and malaria. Dried peel is also burned to repel mosquitoes and as incense. The wood is used for house posts, rafters, tool handles, and small utensils. The bitter seeds have been crushed and mixed with water to make a deworming and ulcer medication.

Lucuma
Pouteria lucuma

Other names
Lucma (Ecuador), rucma (Colombia), mamón (Costa Rica).

Native habitat
Lucuma is native to the highlands of Ecuador, Peru, and the Andean valleys of Bolivia, Ecuador, Chile and Peru. They grow naturally in temperate wet mountain and cloud forest at elevations of 1,500 - 3,000 metres in Peru.

Description
The fruit is round to oval (7-11 cm in diameter), egg shaped, hairless, and green to yellow when mature with a bright yellow , mealy and rather dry pulp. Seeds are dark brown, and glossy. Tastes similar to sweet potato, maple syrup, or butterscotch.

Culinary Use
When eaten raw, the sweet fruit has a mealy and dry texture. In Peru, it is more commonly used as a flavour in ice cream, juice, and milkshakes. The lucuma pulp is sometimes eaten out of the hand but usually used in preserves or stewed as a dessert.

Nutritional value
Lucuma powder is low in sugar, rich in fibre, and a good source of carbohydrates and protein. They are also rich in carotene, vitamin B3 and other B vitamins. It also contains smaller amounts of calcium, phosphorus and iron.

Interesting facts and folklore
Artistic drawings of lúcuma have been found on pottery at burial sites of the native people of coastal Peru. Lucmo seed remnants have been found in Chilca, near Lima dating back to 7500 BC.

Mabolo
Diospyros blancoi

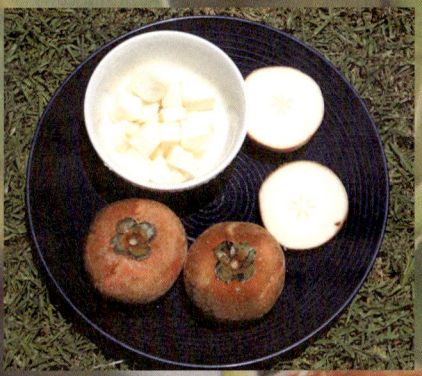

Other names
Velvet apple, velvet persimmon, kamagong, butter fruit, buah lemak, buah mentega.

Native habitat
Native to the Philippines, but it is also native to eastern and southern Taiwan. It is widely distributed in primary and secondary forests at low and medium altitudes in the tropics.

Description
Mabolo produces edible fruit with a fine, velvety, reddish-brown furry covering. The fur is usually rubbed off before eating. Better quality fruit has a creamy-white, soft and mealy flesh with a sweet flavour. The seedless types make better dessert fruits and are moist and sweeter with a cheesy smell.

Culinary Use
Fruit is usually eaten fresh when ripe. Better varieties are rather sweet but often quite dry. They are made into juices, sherbets and table jellies. Fruits should be peeled before eating, and then kept in the refrigerator for a few hours before serving. The flesh can be diced and mixed with other fruits in salads. It can be seasoned with lime or lemon juice and served fresh as dessert.

Nutritional value
Fruits have dietary fibre, vitamins A and C, as well as other minerals. They are a good source of calcium, and potassium and contain B-complex vitamins, iron, and some protein.

Interesting facts and folklore
Mabolo wood is much used in the Philippines in making musical instruments, furniture and exterior work. The Philippine name "mabolo" means hairy, referring to the hairy fruit.

Madrono
Arbutus unedo

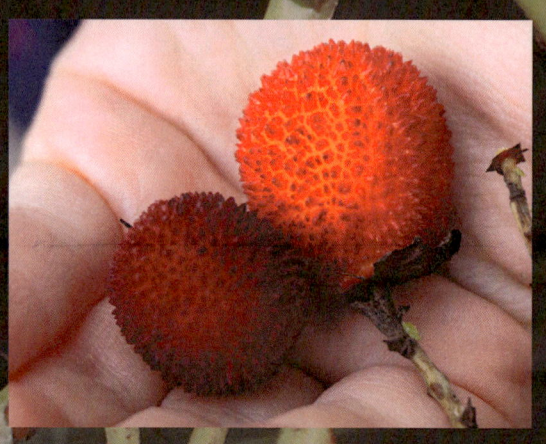

Other names
Strawberry arbutus, Irish strawberry tree, chorleywood arbutus, evergreen strawberry tree.

Native habitat
Madrono is native to the Mediterranean region and western Europe north to western France and Ireland.

Description
Madrono fruits are small (1-3 cm) and round to oval shaped. It has a thin skin with a textured, bumpy surface, covered in soft protrusions. Immature fruits are yellow then ripen to bright red. Madrono's flesh is soft and golden-orange, with many small seeds giving it a soft, gritty texture. The flavour is sweet and sour like a bland peach.

Culinary Use
The pulp is cooked, then sugar and lemon juice is added to make a delicious jam. Madrono fruit is also incorporated into drinks, sauces and jellies.

Nutritional value
Fruits contain phosphorus, potassium, iron and vitamin C.

Interesting facts and folklore
Ancient Romans wove the branches together to make funeral biers, as mourners did for Pallas in Virgil's *Aeneid* (Latin epic poem). In Portugal, madrono is known as *medronho*, and they make a strawberry fruit-based brandy called *aguardente de medronhos*.

Malay apple
Syzygium malaccense

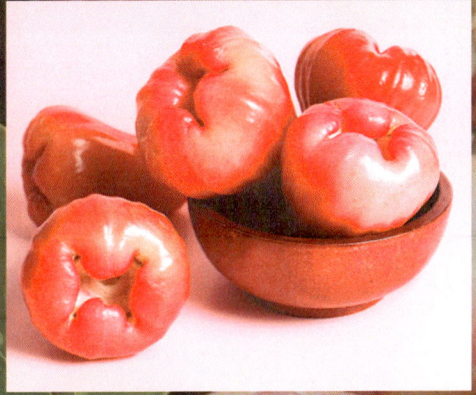

Other names
Pommerac, jambu bol, jambu merah, Malay rose apple, mountain apple, rose apple, Otaheite apple.

Native habitat
Malay apple is native to Vietnam, Malaysia, Indonesia and Australia.

Description
Fleshy dark red, bell shaped berries with white, pink or yellow streaks. Malay apples contain a large round, brown seed. Fruits are crisp, crunchy, juicy and bland but refreshing. They have a thin skin with a mild, slightly acidic, rose flavour.

Culinary Use
The fruits are consumed raw or mixed with other fruits in pies, tarts and custards. They are best eaten as a stewed fruit. Fresh fruits have a short shelf life, 2-3 days. In Puerto Rico they are used in wine making. In Hawaii they are eaten like apples. In Guyana the fruit skins are cooked down to make syrups. Jam is made by stewing the fruit with ginger and brown sugar.

Nutritional value
Malay apples contain fibre, phosphorus, calcium, iron and moderate amounts of phosphorus, calcium and iron.

Interesting facts and folklore
In 1793 Captain Bligh was commissioned to procure many fruits including malay apples from the Pacific Islands and deliver them to Jamaica. A bark infusion was used to treat mouth infections and stomach ache. The leaves have been used to treat skin infections. The roots of the malay apple are used for treating itching and dysentery.

Mamey sapote
Pouteria sapota

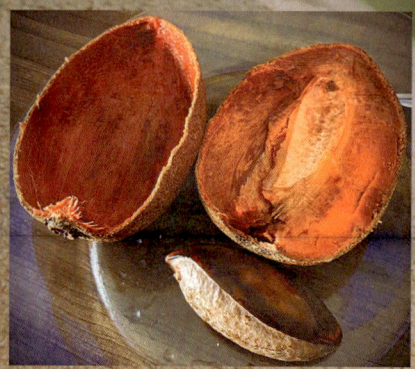

Other names
Red sapote, cico, chico-mamey, green sapote, sapote colorado, zapote colorado, zapote rojo.

Native habitat
The natural habitat is from southern Mexico to Nicaragua. Trees need a humid tropical climate and a forest woodland habitat below 600 metres above sea level.

Description
The fruit is medium to large (8-25 cm), round, with a brown, scaly or scurfy thick skin. The pulp of ripe fruits can be pink, orange, red, or brown in colour, with a soft and smooth, grainy texture, low in fibre. Fruits are very rich and filling, with a sweet, almond or pumpkin flavour. Usually the fruit contains a single, large seed.

Culinary Use
Mamey sapote is eaten fresh out of the hand. Just cut it lengthwise, remove the seed, and eat it like you would avocado by scooping out the flesh. Fresh or frozen pulp is used to make milkshakes, smoothies and ice cream. It is also used in jellies, jams and conserves. Ripe, soft fruits will store well in the refrigerator for several days.

Nutritional value
Fruits are highly nutritious. They contain calcium, phosphorus, iron, magnesium, copper, potassium, vitamin A, C and E, thiamine, riboflavin, and niacin.

Interesting facts and folklore
Relatives in the same family are the sapodilla, caimito, canistel, abiu, and green sapote. When the legendary Cortez and his army travelled 1125 km from Mexico City to Honduras in 1519, at times they relied solely on mamey sapote fruits for food.

Mangaba
Hancornia speciosa

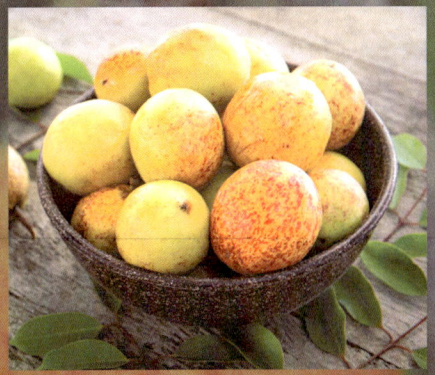

Other names
Mango plum, mangabeira, mangaba rubber tree, mangabinha do norte, mangaba-da-restinga, mangabas, Brazilian apricot.

Native habitat
Native to southern and western South America in Paraguay, Brazil, Bolivia and Peru. It inhabits the scrublands (caatinga and cerrado) and barren lands in central Brazil.

Description
Mangaba fruit is a roundish berry, with a delicate yellow to orange skin, with tiny red spots. The pulp is white, juicy, soft and fleshy with up to 15 disc shaped seeds. It is aromatic with a sweet acid taste.

Culinary use
Fruits are eaten fresh only when fully ripe. Its best to let them fall from the tree to get the best flavour and be free of any latex or bitterness. This leads to a little bruising but are the most sought after in local markets in Brazil. It makes a beautiful marmalade and is used in drinks and sherbets. Frozen pulp has a rich flavour.

Nutritional value
Rich in vitamin C, A, minerals calcium, zinc, phosphorus and iron, proteins and essential oils.

Interesting facts and folklore
In its native home mangaba means "good fruit for eating". Latex from the mangaba tree is used to make rubber. In folk medicine the latex is used for bruises, inflammation, diarrhoea, tuberculosis, ulcers and herpes. An infusion of the leaves has been used to treat menstrual pain.

Mango
Mangifera indica

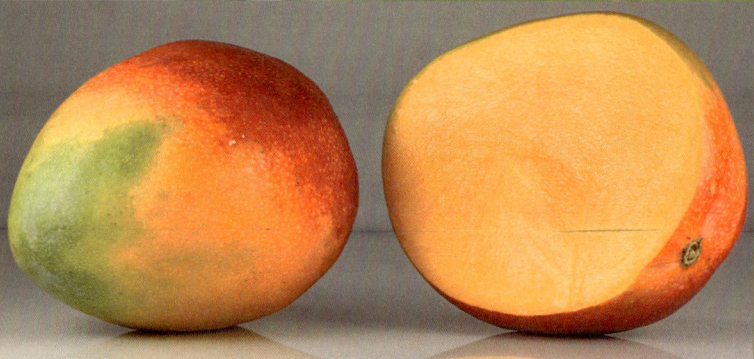

Other names
Mangga, mempelam, pauh, mangas, mempalam.

Native habitat
The natural distribution of mango is in the Indo-Malaysian region, specifically India and Myanmar. Wild populations can be found in the Assam-Chittagong Hills in India.

Description
Mangoes come in many shapes and colours. Some varieties are oval shaped, others round, oblong and some even banana shaped. Fruit colour varies from green to yellow-orange to purple and red. Eating quality is mainly judged on freedom from fibre and lack of turpentine flavour.

Culinary Use
Mangoes are popular eaten fresh as a dessert with cream and ice-cream. They combine well with other fruits in salads, or they may be used in jams, chutneys, pies, cakes, puddings, mousses, sherbets and preserves.

Nutritional value
Rich in vitamin C, vitamin A, potassium, magnesium, phosphorus, and calcium. Good source of dietary fibre. Abundant in antioxidants like polyphenols, flavonoids, and beta-carotene.

Interesting facts and folklore
Mangoes have been cultivated in India for over four thousand years where it has played an important role in Hindu religious ceremony and folklore. The Buddha rested under the shade of a mango tree. In ancient holy books from India mango trees are referred to as being wish-granting trees. Mango is the national fruit of India, Pakistan and the Philippines.

Mangosteen
Garcinia mangostana

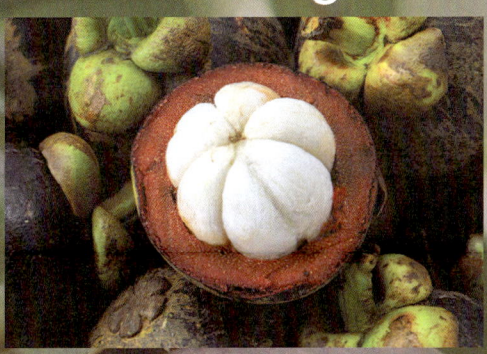

Other names
Queen of fruits, mang cut, mangostan, sementah, san zhu, manggis, manggistan, mangosta, mangostán, mangostana, mangostanier, mangostao, mangostier, meseter.

Native habitat
Mangosteen is native to the tropical jungles of Malaysia, and also to Sumatra.

Description
The mangosteen, also known as the "Queen of Fruits" or purple mangosteen in Southeast Asia, is a tropical fruit prized for its delicious taste and beautiful appearance. The fruit is sweet, tangy, and juicy, with fragrant, fluid-filled segments similar to mandarins. Its inedible rind is deep reddish-purple when ripe. Each fruit has almond-sized seeds, however some are seedless. Mangosteens are typically 2-3 inches in diameter, round or oval-shaped, with a thick, leathery rind.

Culinary Use
Eat mangosteen fresh to best enjoy. Ripe fruit will yield slightly to touch and the rind can be scored around with a sharp knife and the top lifts off easily. Mangosteen sorbet is a delicacy. It can be added to fruit salads, smoothies and yoghurt bowls.

Nutritional value
Mangosteen contains several nutrients with antioxidant capacity, such as vitamin C and manganese. Plus, it provides xanthones which are a unique type of plant compound known to have strong antioxidant properties.

Interesting facts and folklore
Mangosteen rind is very bitter and repels most insects. It is a source of purple dye and is made into kampong toothpaste by charring, pulverising and mixing with a little camphor. The mangosteen was named after a French botanist, Laurent Garcin, who first published a botanical description of this marvellous fruit.

Maprang
Bouea macrophylla

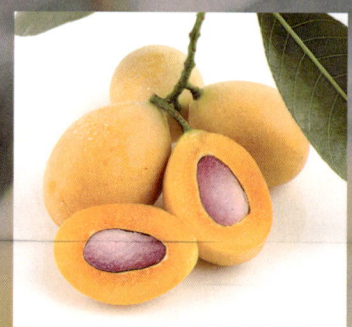

Other names
Gandaria, mango plum, marian plum, egg plum, and plum mango.

Native distribution
The tree is native to North Sumatra, Malaysia and West Java. It grows on tropical lowlands up to an altitude of 850 metres. Trees can tolerate occasional light frosts, and prefer a monsoon climate.

Description
Maprang fruit when immature are green in colour and mature to an orange/yellow. Fruits grow to 5-10 cm in length. The entire fruit, including its skin, is edible. Maprang fruit range from sweet to sour in flavour (depending upon variety) and have a light smell of turpentine. Fruits are soft when ripe and have fibrous mango-like seeds, purple in colour.

Culinary Use
The primary use is as a souring agent, adding a kick to curries, soups, stews, and fish dishes. Pickled or preserved maprang adds a zing to condiments and chutneys. The juice can be used in refreshing drinks, alone or blended. Unripe fruits are used in condiments like sambal and rojak. Eating fruit fresh is best with salt, lime juice, or sugar to balance the acidity.

Nutritional value
Maprang is a great source of vitamin C, calcium, phosphorus, magnesium, iron, thiamine, riboflavin and fibre.

Interesting facts and folklore
Maprang is often used in a dish called Som Chun, a sweet and sour dessert featuring maprang with other fruits like lychee often topped with coconut flakes, peanuts, and ginger. "Som" means sour and "chun" means pungent. It's a unique blend of sweet, salty, and sour flavours.

Maqui berry
Aristotelia chilensis

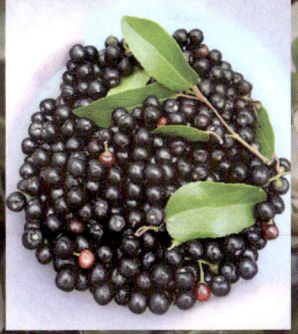

Other names
Chilean wineberry, maquei, quëlón, queldron, koelon, clon.

Native habitat
Maqui (pronounced ma-kee) is native to South America in the Valdivian temperate forests of Chile and adjacent regions of southern Argentina. Maqui is a weedy shrub of cleared forests and waste ground, growing in moist, humus rich soils on lower mountain slopes by rivers between latitudes 31 and 40° south in Chile and Argentina.

Description
The small, purple-black, pea sized berries contain 4 to 8 angled seeds. The fruit that tastes like bilberries or blackberries, The berries of A. chilensis are collected from wild plants in summer each year by Mapuche families in Patagonia. Berries are sweet and refreshing, with a slight astringency.

Culinary Use
Fruits are eaten fresh or dried for winter use. A popular drink *chicha de maqui* is made by simply mashing fruit and mixing with water and the liquid is drawn off and consumed. Berries are dipped in boiling water to loosen the skin, before being dried, ground into a powder, extracted and pressed. It is exported in this form for the production of natural colourings.

Nutritional value
The maqui berry is considered to be one of the highest food sources of antioxidants, in particular anthocyanins, which targets and neutralises free radicals. They are high in dietary fibre, calcium, iron, magnesium, vitamins A and C.

Interesting facts and folklore
Berries are used to treat or prevent dry eyes, lung damage, and diabetes. Mapuches historically gave Maqui berries to their warriors to improve their strength and stamina.

Matisia
Quararibea cordata

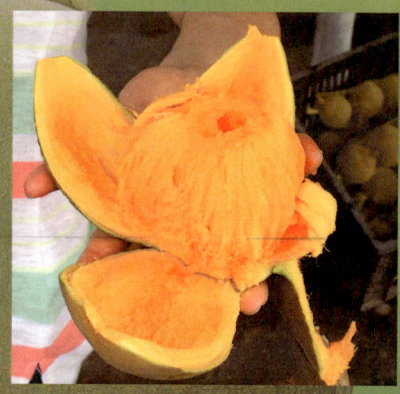

Other names
South American sapote, chupa chupa.

Native habitat
Matisia is native to the Amazon rainforest vegetation in Brazil, Colombia, Ecuador, and Peru, Venezuela. It inhabits the hot, humid lowland forest of lower Andes.

Description
Matisia fruits are large (10-15cm) round to oval or elliptical and have a rind that is thick, leathery, and greenish brown. The orange- yellow fibrous flesh is soft, juicy and sweet with a flavour reminiscent of pumpkin, mango or rockmelon. There are 2-5 seeds with long fibres that permeate the flesh similar to a mango seed. Fruits are picked when a light coloured halo appears around the stem end. Don't wait for fruits to drop as they are rotten by then. Fruits soften and are ripe in 3-4 days after at room temperatures. Better varieties have shrivelled seeds and less fibrous flesh.

Culinary Use
These fruits are typically consumed fresh by hand or juiced. Some better types have little fibre, perfect for making refreshing fruit juices. They also make great desserts such as ice cream and fruit smoothies.

Nutritional value
Contains calcium and phosphorus for bones and teeth, and vitamin C for immune support. Good amounts of fibre and vitamin A, carotene.

Interesting facts and folklore
The common name chupa chupa is derived from the Spanish word chupa, to suck, describing how the pulp has to be sucked to separate it from the seeds.

Miracle fruit
Synsepalum dulcificum

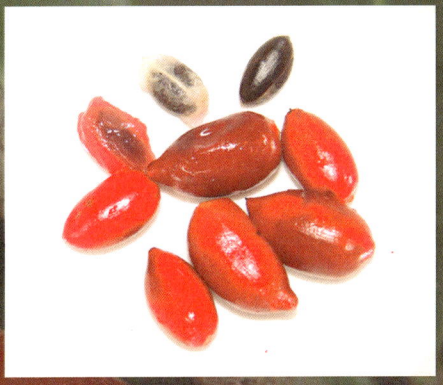

Other names
Miracle berry, miraculous berry, sweet berry, African sweet berry, asaa, agbayun, taami, ledidi.

Native habitat
Miracle fruit comes from the hot, tropical lowlands of Western and Central Tropical Africa.

Description
The plant bears a profusion of small, bright red, olive shaped fruits, with a sweet white flesh with a single smooth and shiny seed. The fruits taper to a slight point and are 1-2 cm long. They ripen from green to bright red. The inner translucent flesh is mildly sweet but virtually tasteless.

Culinary Use
The berry is high in miraculin, a glycoprotein molecule, which binds to taste receptors that are near the sweet receptor sites in your mouth, sweetening the taste of sour or acidic foods, such as vinegar or lemons. At the same time it doesn't affect the taste of sweet foods.

Nutritional value
Miracle fruit berries are a great sources of Vitamins C, A, and E and essential amino acids.

Interesting facts and folklore
Miracle fruits act on the sour receptors of the taste buds turning all sour tasting foods sweet. Just a small amount of each tiny fruit is sufficient and the effect lasts for 30 minutes or more. In Ghana, the miracle fruit is used to sweeten sour foods and beverages, such as kenkey, koko, and palm wine.

Mountain soursop
Annona montana

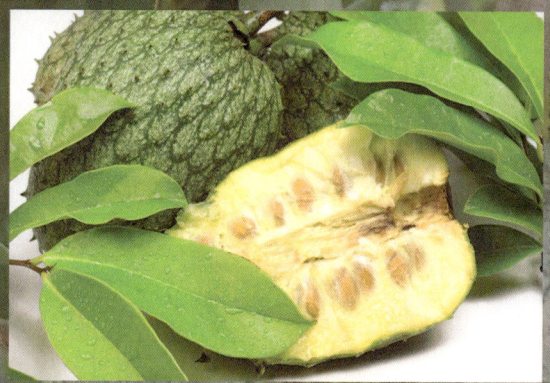

Other names
Custard apple, cherimoya, guanabana, soursop, mountain sop.

Native habitat
The mountain soursop is home to Brazil, Bolivia, Peru, Ecuador, Colombia, Venezuela, Panama, Costa Rica and the Caribbean. In its native habitat it grows at altitudes from sea level to 650 metres.

Description
The fruit is almost round with a dark green skin covered with short, fleshy, prickly spines. The skin turns a paler colour when ripe. It is not considered as nice as its relative the soursop, but it is more cold tolerant which makes it useful to grow in subtropical areas down to -2 deg C. The fruits are about 15 centimetres (5.9 in) long. Mountain soursops have a lemon yellow coloured fibrous flesh. It is aromatic with a sour to bitter taste and contains lots of brown, plump seeds.

Culinary Use
Fruits are eaten fresh and made into juices. Fully ripe fruit is eaten fresh for dessert or mixed with ice cream and milk to make a milkshake. Immature fruits are cooked as a vegetable in soups. Ripe fruits are quite perishable and storage life is short.

Nutritional value
Mountain soursops have high levels of vitamin A and C, beta-carotene, and are a good source of potassium and magnesium.

Interesting facts and folklore
The scientific name *Montana* means, "coming from the mountains". The fruit, seeds, bark, leaves, and roots have all been used to treat asthma and bronchitis, inflammation, diabetes, hypertension and worms.

Nance fruit
Brysonima crassifolia

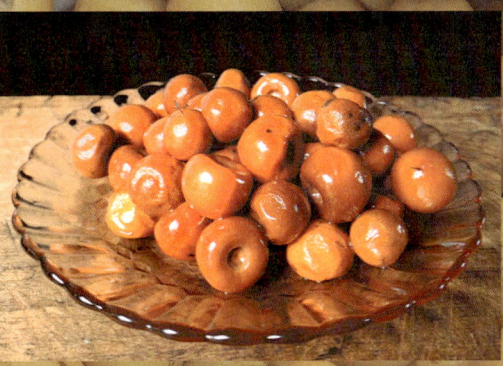

Other names
Golden spoon, wild cherry, maricao cimun, craboo, changunga, muruci, nancite, savanna serrette, hogberry, nanche.

Native habitat
Native to Central America, South America, and Mexico. It is found wild in tropical deciduous forests and the Amazonian savannas up to an elevation of 1800 metres.

Description
The small, round, sweet bright yellow fruits (1-2 cm wide) resemble a cherry and have a distinct smell and flavour resembling cheese or a mix of banana, lychee and pear. They are thin-skinned with a creamy, white, juicy, and oily flesh with 1-3 white seeds.

Culinary Use
Nance fruits are eaten raw or cooked as dessert. Nance fruits cooked in sugar and water make a candy *dulce de nance*. Nance fruits are also used to prepare soda drinks, ice cream and juice, cookies, cakes, sorbets, jellies, liqueurs, jams, nectars, and pickles.

Nutritional value
Vitamin C (60% DV), dietary fibre, vitamin K and E, manganese, potassium, iron, magnesium, calcium and copper.

Interesting facts and folklore
In Panama, the wood from the tree is used as an aromatic in smoking and grilling. The leaves and stems can stun fish and local tribes have traditionally used these to harvest fish. The bark is rich in tannins and is used as a treatment for gastrointestinal problems, and snakebites. It is also applied to skin infections and ulcers. A dessert prepared with sugar and flour is known as pesada de nance.

Naranjilla
Solanum quitoense

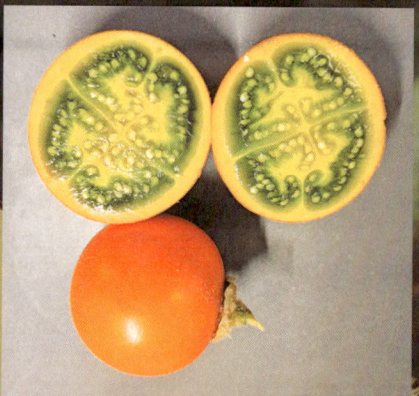

Other names
Lulo, quito orange, golden fruit of the Andes, naranjina, toronjita, lulito.

Native habitat
Naranjilla is native to the subtropical regions of the Andes of Ecuador, to Peru, and to southern Columbia.

Description
Ripe fruit has a citrus flavour, sometimes described as a combination of rhubarb and lime. The juice of the naranjilla is green and is often used as a juice or for a drink called lulada. The hairs on the skin of the fruit are rubbed off before the fruit is eaten. The bright orange-yellow fruits are small (4-6 cm), round to oval, and have a thick peel. Inside is a delicious juicy, acidic, green to yellowish pulp with a pineapple-lemon flavour.

Culinary Use
Naranjilla fruits are added as flavouring for native dishes, ice cream, sherbets, and other desserts. In Colombia, fruits are used as a base in a drink called lulada, made with mashed naranjilla, lime juice, water, sugar, and ice.

Nutritional value
Fruits contain high amounts of fibre, calcium , and vitamins A and C, zinc, magnesium, thiamine, niacin, vitamin K, and riboflavin.

Interesting facts and folklore
Naranjilla (pronounced na-ran-hee-ya) means "little orange" in Spanish. They have been described as "the golden fruit of the Andes." Naranjilla fruits are believed to detox the body, promote digestion, and even improve skin complexion.

Otaheite gooseberry
Phyllanthus acidus

Other names
Barbados gooseberry, Malay gooseberry, Indian gooseberry, wild lime, star gooseberry, wei-zha-mu (Chinese), grosella, ronde, birambi, guinda.

Native habitat
Otaheite gooseberries are a tropical plant that were previously thought to be native to Madagascar but originally they inhabited north-eastern Brazil. It is a shrub or small tree that grows primarily in the wet tropics.

Description
The small edible gooseberries are pale yellow-green or creamy-white, waxy, juicy and crisp, with a very sour taste. There are 4 to 6 seeds contained in a hard stone in the middle of each fruit. The fruit grow on trunk and branches, densely clustered along the limbs and dangling from young twigs.

Culinary Use
It is a main ingredient in sweet relishes and preserves in its native habitat of India and Madagascar. Fruits are used to make vinegar as well as eaten raw, soaked in vinegar-salt solution and sold along the roadside. The sour berries are candied as well and stored in jars with syrup. They are used to make fruit juice with plenty of sugar added. In Thailand the berries are used as an ingredient to make Som tam, a green salad.

Nutritional value
Rich in vitamin C, traces of vitamin B, and minerals iron, calcium, manganese, potassium, and zinc.

Interesting facts and folklore
The peppered leaves are used to treat sciatica and rheumatism. The fruit is also used as a laxative. In India the bark from the roots is used as a tanning agent.

Panama berry
Muntingia calabura

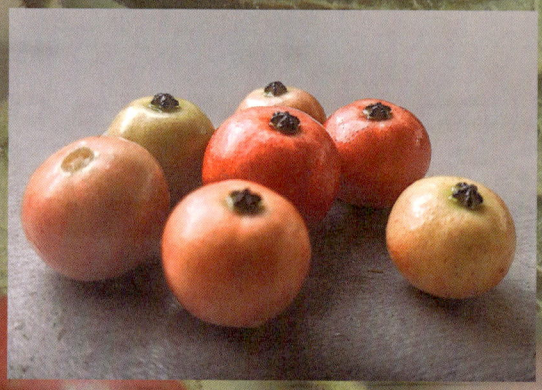

Other names
Strawberry tree, Singapore cherry, calabur tree, West Indian cherry, Japanese cherry, Jamaica cherry.

Native habitat
Native to southern Mexico, the Caribbean, Central America, and western South America to Bolivia and Argentina. It is found growing in tropical climates in well drained soils in the lowlands to a height of 600 to 1000 metres. It is an invasive species in its wild habitat.

Description
Panama berry is a small red fruit (1.5cm) that has a very sweet tasting, light brown, juicy pulp with thousands of very fine seeds that are unnoticeable when eaten, and a flavour similar to caramel or figs. They are green when immature and ripen to a red colour (yellow type as well).

Culinary Use
Ripe berries are mainly eaten fresh out of the hand. It can be made into jams and cooked in tarts and pies.

Nutritional value
Good levels of vitamin C and K, as well as calcium, iron, and potassium.

Interesting facts and folklore
Tea can be infused from the leaves of the tree, and the flowers are said to have antiseptic and antispasmodic properties and have been used to treat headaches. A tough, pliable, cord can be made from the tree bark for fastenings and basket weaving. Trees are planted along river banks in Brazil as fish are attracted to the fallen fruits.

Papaya
Carica papaya

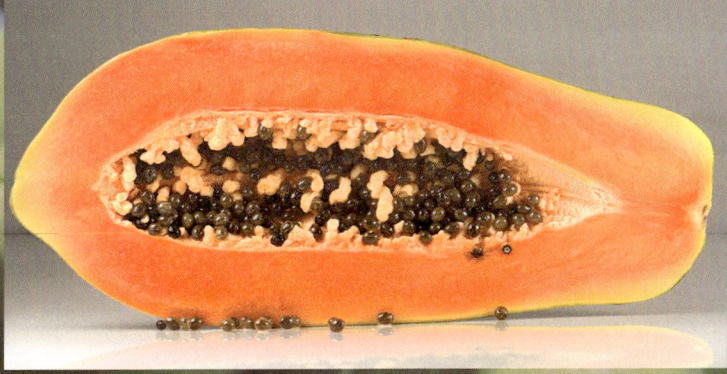

Other names
Paw paw, tree melon, papaw, papita (in Spanish), mamao (in Portuguese), du du, kates, and pepe.

Native habitat
Papaya is native to the tropical, lowland regions of Central America and southern Mexico.

Description
The papaya fruit is large (15-50cm), melon-like, round to cylindrical in shape, and sometimes weighing as much as 10 kg. It ripens to an orange- yellow colour with a smooth skin. The juicy, orange or red flesh is sweet with a musky flavour. The central cavity contains numerous round, often wrinkled, black seeds.

Culinary Use
Papaya is used in salads, pies, sherbets, juices, and confections. It is also used to make jams, jellies, and ice cream. In the West Indies the unripe fruit is cooked like the vegetable, squash.

Nutritional value
Papaya is a good source of calcium and excellent source of vitamins C, A. It also contains folate, magnesium, copper, pantothenic acid, fibre, B vitamins, alpha and beta-carotene, lutein and zeaxanthin, vitamin E, K, calcium, potassium, and lycopene (excellent antioxidant).

Interesting facts and folklore
Carica papaya has potent antioxidant properties. Unripe fruit contains a digesting enzyme known as papain. The juice from the unripe fruit was used by the Central American Indians as a remedy for indigestion and to tenderise meat.

Passionfruit
Passiflora edulis

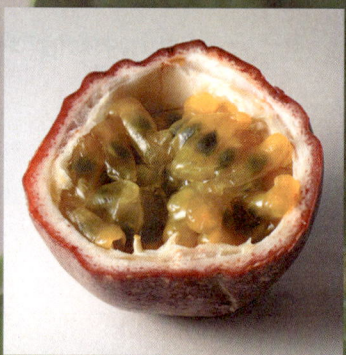

Other names
Grenadelle, grenadine, passionflower, purple granadilla, purple passion fruit.

Native habitat
Passionfruit are native to the region of southern Brazil through Paraguay to northern Argentina.

Description
Passion fruits are a round to oval berry. They are purple, red or gold with a tough, smooth rind, ranging in colour from dark-purple with fine white specks, to light-yellow. Under the rind is a cavity filled with an aromatic mass of sacs filled with orange, pulpy juice and as many small, hard, dark-brown or black seeds. The flavour of the pulp is similar to guava, with a sweet to acid taste.

Culinary Use
Fruits are ripe when they change colour from green to purple, and if left on the vine the skins begin to wrinkle. Pick them plump before they wrinkle and let them ripen in the fruit bowl for a few days for full sweetness. Passionfruit juice can be boiled down and used in making sauce, candy, ice cream, sherbet, cake icing and filling, meringue, or in cocktails.

Nutritional value
Passionfruit are a good source of fibre, rich in antioxidants, potassium, iron, vitamin C, and provitamin A. They are also rich in beneficial plant compounds, including carotenoids and polyphenols.

Interesting facts and folklore
Catholic missionaries thought the flower crowns represented the crown of thorns. The stamens the five wounds and the ten petals the ten fruitful apostles. This gave rise to its common name, passionfruit.

Peach palm
Bactris gasipaes

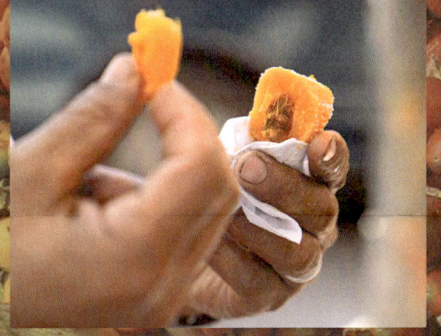

Other names
Pejibaye, macana, pupunha, pejivalle, chontaduro, pewa palm, pijuayo, chonta de castilla, tembe, siri, ziri, uwi, pisbae.

Native habitat
South western Amazon basin in what is now northern Bolivia, south eastern Peru and western Brazil, although the exact origin is unknown. In the wild it is found along river beds and in the primary forest.

Description
Peach palm is a stone fruit with edible pulp surrounding the single seed. The rind of the fruit can be red, yellow, or orange when ripe, depending on variety. The fruits grow in large bunches of 80 to 100 stone fruits. The skin is smooth, thin, slightly wrinkled, and greasy. Underneath, the flesh has a dense, starchy consistency with a fibrous texture. There is a small, brown seed.

Culinary Use
Fruits are typically boiled in salt water and pork fat for 60 minutes and when cool the skin is peeled, and the seed is removed. They are then halved and served with mayonnaise. It can be cooked to make cake, muffins and chontaduro chips.

Nutritional value
Fruits are a good source of fibre and provide some vitamins A, C, and E, which are antioxidants. The fruits also contain minerals, including magnesium, phosphorus, zinc, copper, iron, and calcium. They are an excellent supply of carbohydrates, proteins, fatty acids and amino acids.

Interesting facts and folklore
Peach-palms are also cultivated for the heart of palm, and the trunk can make valuable timber.

Persimmon
Diospyros kaki

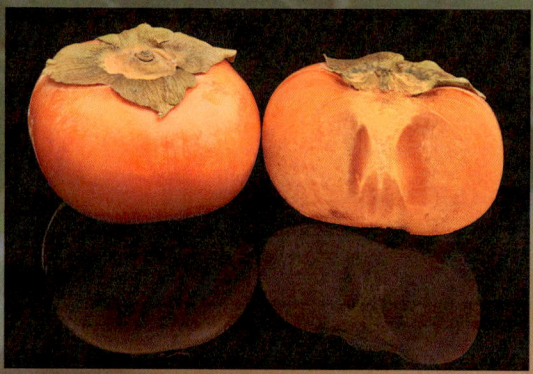

Other names
Oriental persimmon, Japanese persimmon, kaki (Japanese), sharon fruit, Chinese persimmon, American persimmon, date-plum, Japan apple, kaki persimmon.

Native habitat
The persimmon originated in eastern Asia, and native cultivars are scattered from temperate to subtropical regions of China.

Description
Fruits are round to oval with a sweet, slightly tangy with a soft, sometimes fibrous texture. Ripe fruit has a thick pulpy jelly encased in a waxy, thin-skinned shell. The smooth, shiny, thin skin ranges in colour from yellow to red-orange. As the fruit reaches maturity it softens up similar to a kiwifruit.

Culinary Use
There are two fruiting types, astringent and non astringent. Astringent fruit must be left until they soften up due to their tannins, whereas non astringent persimmons can be eaten crunchy like an apple straight from the tree. Eaten fresh they are delicious, they can also be frozen, dried, and made into beer, cider or wine. They are used in pies, salads, juices, ice cream, and dressings.

Nutritional value
Persimmons have a high content of the carotenoids beta-cryptoxanthin, beta-carotene, and zeaxanthin. They also contain potassium, manganese, and vitamins A, C and B.

Interesting facts and folklore
Persimmon leaves are used to wrap sushi. In autumn, after the trees have lost their leaves, families and farmers from the rural areas collect persimmons and hang them to dry.

Pitaya
Selenicereus undatus

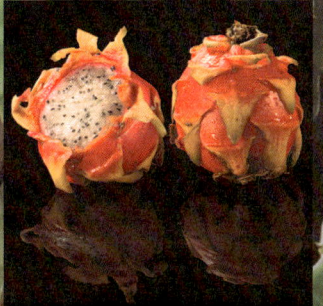

Other names
White dragon fruit, pitaya blanca (in Spanish), dragonfruit, thanh long trắng (in Vietnamese), huo long guo (in Chinese), strawberry pear, night-blooming cereus, moonflower cactus.

Native habitat
Pitaya is native to the tropical and subtropical regions of Central America. Its habitat includes southern Mexico, Honduras, Guatemala, El Salvador and Costa Rica.

Description
Pitaya fruits are oblong to oval in shape and may grow up to 12.5cm. They are dragon-like with thick red bracteoles (leaflike structures) outside and they have a sweet, soft, delicious and fleshy fruit inside. The white flesh is speckled with tiny black, edible seeds, mild in flavour. Pitaya fruit has a taste similar to a blend of kiwifruit, pear, and watermelon.

Culinary Use
Pitaya is delicious served chilled, either sliced or eaten with a spoon. They make sauces, sorbets, and delicious breakfast bowls. If you puree them and freeze them you can blend into smoothies or drinks. You can store your fresh pitaya fruits for up to a few days in the fruit bowl at room temperature. You can mix fruit in a bowl with other tropicals like papaya, pineapple, and kiwifruit.

Nutritional value
Pitaya fruits are rich in antioxidants such as flavonoids, phenolic acid, and betacyanin. They also contain prebiotics and are high in vitamin C, magnesium, calcium, iron and fibre but low in calories.

Interesting facts and folklore
The cactus tree bears stunning white, fragrant flowers that only bloom for one night. In the tropics, the flowers depend on pollination by bats.

Pomegranate
Punica granatum

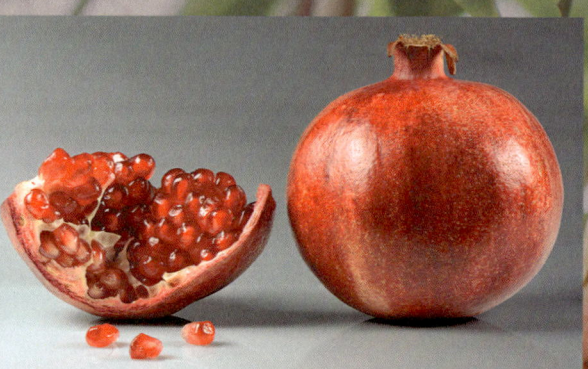

Other names
Wine apples, grenade, delima, Carthaginian apple.

Native habitat
Pomegranate is native to a region from Iran to northern India. The trees will grow in a wide range of climates, however the highest quality fruit is produced in areas where the fruit ripens under high temperatures and a dry atmosphere.

Description
Each fruit contains hundreds of seeds, surrounded by red, pink or pale yellow flesh. The flesh is enclosed by an astringent, inedible pith. The seeds of pomegranates have a sweet and tart taste. Red fruits are the most popular, but they can also be found in white, pink, yellow, and purple. The round, leathery skinned fruits are the size of an apple.

Culinary Use
Pomegranates are used in baking, cooking, juice blends, meal garnishes, smoothies, and cocktails and wine.

Nutritional value
The pomegranate is one of the healthiest fruits, with a high concentration of antioxidants. They are rich in vitamin C and fibre.

Interesting facts and folklore
The plant was first grown around 3000 BC or earlier by the ancient Persians. The name pomegranate is derived from the Latin words "pomum granatum," which means the "apple with many seeds." Some believe that the forbidden fruit eaten by Eve in Eden was a pomegranate, not an apple. Pomegranates symbolised the afterlife and were given as offerings and placed in tombs and graves to send the departed on their journey.

Pomelo
Citrus maxima

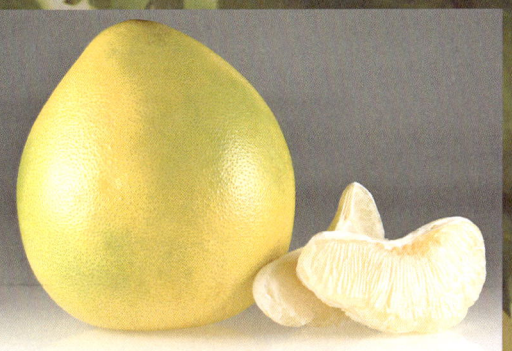

Other names
Pomello, pummelo, pamplemousse, jabong (Hawaii), shaddock, limau bali, limau besar, limau betawi.

Native habitat
Pomelos originated in a geographical arc from Malaysia through Indonesia to Papua New Guinea. Plants prefer warm tropical to subtropical climates with abundant rainfall.

Description
Pomelos are the largest of citrus fruits, round to pear-shaped with a thick, textured rind ranging from green to bright yellow. Beneath the peel and bitter white pith are the juicy segments of flesh, varying in colour and sweetness/tartness depending on the variety. The pulp segments are either white, yellow or pink and shell out easily from the thick rind. Fruit taste is reminiscent of grapefruit, but sweet instead of sour with less juice.

Culinary Use
The flesh and juice of pomelo are consumed, the rind is used for preserves or candied, and in Brazil, the thick skin is used for a sweet conserve. Pomelos are commonly eaten as desserts, sometimes with sugar or salt, and can be made into salads. A pink beverage is made from pomelo and pineapple juice.

Nutritional value
Pomelos are rich in vitamin C, copper for a healthy nervous system, potassium for fluid balance, and smaller amounts of phosphorus, fibre, and calcium.

Interesting facts and folklore
Pomelos have been cultivated in China for centuries. They are traditionally eaten during the Lunar New Year as the fruit is said to represent prosperity and status.

Prickly pear
Opuntia humifusa

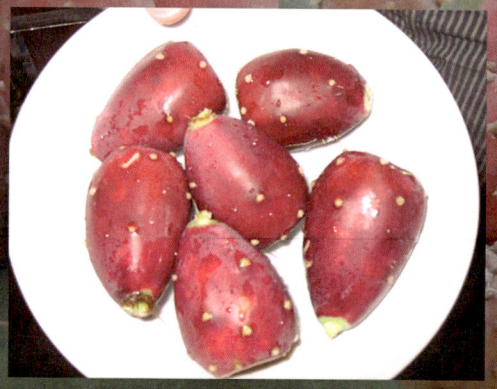

Other names
Devils tongue, Eastern prickly pear, nopal cactus, paddle cactus.

Native habitat
Prickly pear is native to the eastern USA from Massachusetts to Florida and in scattered areas of the midwest. *Opuntia humifusa* is found growing naturally in open, dry and arid areas, often on rock or poor, hungry soils. It is commonly seen by roadsides, rocky outcrops, cliffs and prairie in well drained soils.

Description
Prickly pear has juicy green, red, purple, or yellow-orange egg-shaped fruits that grow on the edge of the flat pads. As the fruit matures it changes colour from the unripe green. They are covered in glochids (hair like splinters, spiny bristles) that are very painful if they lodge in your skin and so hard to see.

Culinary Use
You can eat prickly pear flesh raw or cooked. Wear thick gloves to twist the fruits off the pads and rub off the glochids. Peel back the skin and you are left with the pear shaped fruit.You can scoop out the pulp and strain the seeds out to make candies, jellies and syrups. The flesh has a sweet taste similar to that of a watermelon.

Nutritional value
Prickly pear is a good source of dietary fibre and antioxidants, magnesium, potassium, calcium and vitamin C.

Interesting facts and folklore
Native Americans ate the fruits (fresh, cooked or dried for winter), roasted the pads as a vegetable, and used the sap for certain medicinal applications.

Pulasan
Nephelium ramboutan

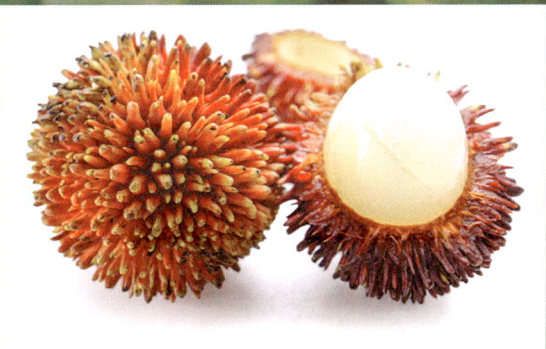

Other names
Kapulasan, capulassan, pulassan, bulala, nephelium ramboutan-ake, purasan, rambutan paroh.

Native habitat
Pulasan is native to Borneo and Peninsular Malaysia. It is very closely related to rambutan. Pulasan grows best in the lowland humid tropics at an elevation below 600 metres, not tolerating frost. Trees are found on river banks but rarely in swamps, usually on sand or clay.

Description
Pulasan fruit has a thicker rind and is generally juicier and more acidic than its close relative the rambutan, however there are many wild types with differing characteristics. Twist the fruit open to eat the white, succulent flesh. Mostly eaten out of hand, it can also be used in jams and jellies. The fruit is round, dark red, fleshy, and with a thick and leathery rind similar to that of rambutan but has no hairy spines. The seed is usually round or oblong, and light brown. They are edible raw and have a flavour similar to that of almonds.

Culinary Use
Pulasan fruit is eaten raw or cooked then made into jams and fruit desserts. The seeds are roasted and used in the preparation of a cocoa drink.

Nutritional value
Pulasan is a good source of vitamin C, calcium and iron. Fruits have antibacterial, antioxidant, and anticancer properties.

Interesting facts and folklore
The leaves and roots have been used as poultices and to treat fever. An oil is obtained from the seed and used in cooking and lamps.

Rambai
Baccaurea motleyana

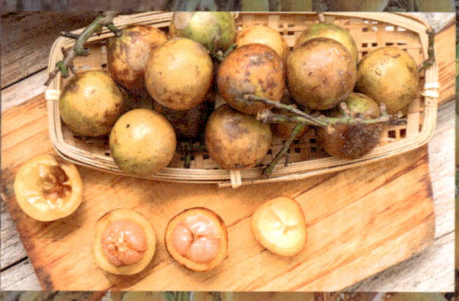

Other names
Red rambai, rambi , mafia-farang (Thai), white rambai, lotkon, bhabhi (Bangladesh), rambe, kepundung, and menteng.

Native habitat
Rambai are believed to have originated in Kalimantan, Java, Sumatra, Bali, and Peninsula Malaysia. Trees thrive in the tropical rainforests of Malaysia,Thailand, Indonesia (including Sumatra and Borneo),and the Philippines.

Description
Fruits are small and round and have a thin, smooth, velvety skin that changes from green to yellow, brown, or pink when ripe. They grow in clusters on thin branches or trunks. Flavour is sweet-tart or sweet-sour, sometimes compared to mango, pineapple, and banana. Each small brown seed is encased in a sweet, edible, white to purple flesh.

Culinary Use
Rambai fruit is eaten raw. Just peel them and suck the flesh off the seed. Make them into drinks or they are sometimes pickled and served with curries. The fruit can be incorporated into jams, jellies, syrups, dried snacks and wines. Unripe rambai can be used in chutneys. Blend rambai into juices or smoothies. Fruits are cooked in soups, stews, curries, and desserts. Delicious in sorbets, and ice creams. Rambai complements fish, prawns, and poultry.

Nutritional value
The fruits of B. *motleyana* are a good source of vitamin C and B12, phosphorus, potassium and magnesium, and fibres. They also contain bioactive compounds such as phenolic acids, flavonoids, carotenoids, and terpenes.

Interesting facts and folklore
Traditionally, an extract from its bark is used to treat sore eyes. Extracts of rambai peel have been found to possess antimicrobial properties.

Rambutan
Nephelium lappaceum

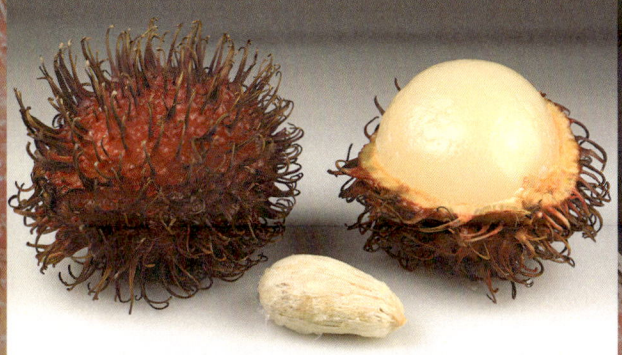

Other names
Hairy lychee, ramboutan, ramboutanier, ramboostan, shao tzu, Ngoh, phruan, chom chom, hong mao dan.

Native habitat
The rambutan is native to Southeast Asia. They are home to the lowland humid forests of Malaysia and Indonesia.

Description
The name rambutan is derived from the Malay word *rambut* meaning 'hair' referring to the thick covering of soft red, yellow or pink spines on the fruits. They are typically small, oval to round, 3-5 cm in diameter, and grow in loose, hanging clusters of 10 to 20 fruits. Inside the skin is the sweet, white translucent flesh which has a mild sub acidic flavour. It is very refreshing, similar to lychees. There is a single fibrous seed which is sometimes roasted.

Culinary Use
The fruit of the rambutan tree may be eaten raw by removing the peel, eating the pulp, and discarding the seed. Rambutan is most often used in desserts, such as sorbets and puddings, but also in curries and savoury dishes. The flavour is similar to lychee and goes well with other tropical fruits.

Nutritional value
Fruits contain vitamin C, good amounts of fibre, copper, iron, phosphorus, manganese, and magnesium.

Interesting facts and folklore
Every year in August the Surat Thani rambutan fair is held to celebrate this wonderful fruit. The first rambutan tree was planted in Surat Thani in 1926, and this fair celebrates this delicious fruit, which now grows widely in the area.

Red mombin
Spondias purpurea

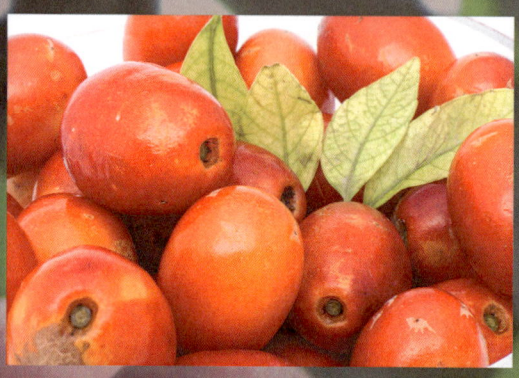

Other names
Red mombin, Spanish plum, purple mombin, Jamaica plum, hog plum, jocote (derived from the Nahuatl word xocotl, meaning "any kind of sour or acidic fruit") jobillo.

Native habitat
Red mombin is native to tropical regions of the Americas, from Mexico to northern Colombia and the southwest Caribbean Islands. They grow wild in thickets and open forest, often in secondary growth, common in fencerows, pastures from sea level to elevations of about 1700 metres.

Description
Red mombin fruits are small (3-5 cm), oval shaped and plum-like with a thin, waxy and glossy skin often with light brown speckles. They vary in colour from purple, bright-red, to yellow sometimes. The flesh is aromatic, yellow, fibrous, very juicy, with a rich sweet sour flavour. Within the flesh is a large, inedible seed.

Culinary Use
Ripe red mombin fruits are commonly eaten out-of-hand or they are stewed whole, with sugar, and eaten as dessert. They can be preserved by boiling and drying. The strained juice from cooked fruit makes a jelly and is also used for making wine and vinegar. They can also be made into jams, chutney, boiled or dried fruits.

Nutritional value
Vitamin C and A, phosphorus, calcium, and magnesium.

Interesting facts and folklore
A fruit decoction is used to bathe wounds and heal mouth sores. A syrup from the fruit is taken to relieve chronic diarrhoea. The tree leaves are fed to cattle and the fruits are fed to hogs.

Rollinia
Rollinia mucosa

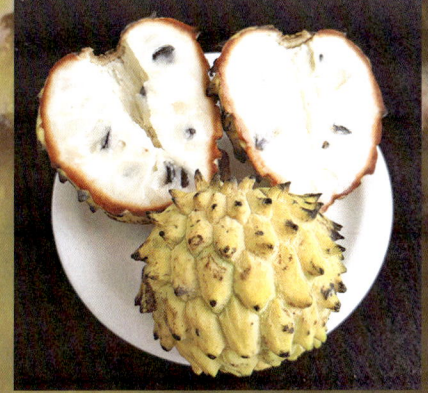

Other names
Biriba, wild sugar apple, arazá, fruta da condessa, jaca de pobre, araticu, condongo, lemon meringue pie fruit, Amazon custard apple.

Native habitat
Rollinia comes from the western Amazon basin of Brazil. It is found growing wild in northern Brazil along the banks of the Amazon river. It is also found in its natural state in Guiana, southern Mexico, Peru, and northern Argentina.

Description
Rollinia is a large, conical or heart shaped fruit. This wonderful fruit turns from green to yellow when ripe. It has a white, pyramidal shaped segments of flesh containing numerous black, inedible seeds. Its surface is bumpy and covered with soft spines which bruise and blacken with excessive handling. Flesh is slightly sweet and tastes similar to lemon sherbet or lemon meringue pie.

Culinary Use
Fruit is usually eaten fresh or used raw. Just cut the fruit in half and scoop out the delicious pulp, discarding the seeds. The skin of ripe fruit peels away easily. Mix with other fresh fruits in an exotic dessert. The pulp can be used to make jams or jellies or pureed and mixed with milk for smoothies. It can be cooked into pies, cakes, or souffles.

Nutritional value
Rollinia fruit is high in calcium and phosphorus, as well as vitamin C and iron.

Interesting facts and folklore
Trees have hardwood that is used to make boat masts and ribs for canoes.

Santol
Sandoricum koetjape

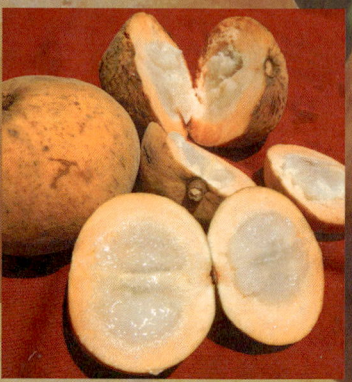

Other names
Cotton fruit, sentul, kechapi, kecapi, kelampu, ketjape, ketuat, lolly fruit, ranggu, yellow or red santol.

Native habitat
Santol is found growing naturally in tropical regions of Malaysia, Cambodia, and Laos. In its native forest habitat santol is a lofty tree growing as high as 30 or 50 metres with a smooth, straight trunk. The dark green leaves turn to some beautiful autumn shades of red or yellow as the trees become semi deciduous.

Description
The fruit are orange-yellow, round to oval and flattened in shape. The skins are tough, wrinkled, leathery with a slight fuzz. There are red or yellow fruit types. The soft, white, translucent flesh is juicy, thirst quenching and in some varieties has a rather peachy aroma. Fruits have a sweet and sour flavour.

Culinary Use
Santol fruits are eaten fresh or cooked into candies, jellies, jams and a syrup used as a topping over ice cream.

Nutritional value
Santol is a good source of iron, vitamin C and fibre. Also calcium, phosphorus, potassium and vitamin B.

Interesting facts and folklore
Santol has been used in natural medications. The bark, leaves, roots and fruits used in treating skin allergies, infections and stomach digestion. Fruits are believed to reduce inflammation. The large seeds are inedible and dangerous if swallowed as they can cause intestinal blockages.

Sapodilla
Manilkara zapote

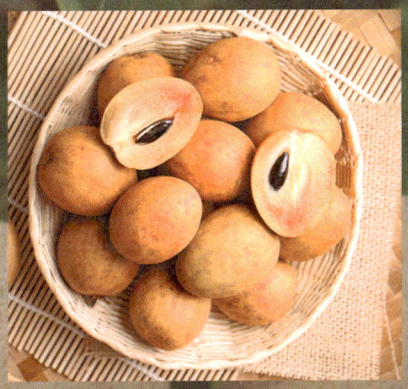

Other names
Sapote, chicozapote, chicoo, chicle (referring to the latex extracted from the tree), naseberry, nispero, soapapple, buah chiku, chiko, and korob.

Native habitat
Central America, Mexico, Panama and the West Indies in lowland and coastal forests, They are found in moist, hot tropical climates below 900 metres.

Description
The fruit is a large berry (4-8cm), round to oval shape with a russet brown, thin skin somewhat resembling a kiwifruit and a very sweet, yellow brown flesh, soft, melting and aromatic with a malty, caramel or brown sugar taste. There are 6-12 shiny brown or black seeds present.

Culinary Use
Sapodillas may be eaten fresh out of the hand by scooping out the flesh from the thin skin or made into sherbets, custards and ice cream. Blend the flesh with orange juice and cream to make a dessert sauce. Pulp can be cooked with ginger and lime juice and can be used as a filling for pies and tarts. Best to eat sapodillas when fully ripe so that they have lost their astringency.

Nutritional value
High in vitamin C, fibre, copper, and good amounts of potassium, magnesium, iron, folate, and vitamin B5.

Interesting facts and folklore
The sapodilla was discovered during the Spanish explorations where it was referred to by the Aztecs as chikl . It's been cultivated in Guatemala and Belize for a white latex (chicle) which was used as a base for chewing gum.

Sea grape
Coccoloba uvifera

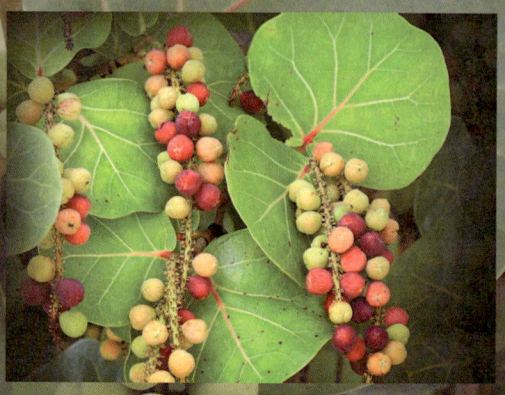

Other names
Bay grape, common sea grape, Jamaican kino, platterleaf, seaside grape, beach grape, uva de playa (in Spanish), coccoloba, sea raisin, shore grape, raisin de mer (in French) kurena (in Taino, an indigenous language).

Native habitat
Sea grape is native to coastal beaches throughout tropical America and the Caribbean, including central & southern Florida, the Bahamas, the Greater and Lesser Antilles, and Bermuda.

Description
Sea grape bears green fruit (2 cm) in large clusters like grapes. The fruit gradually ripens to a purplish colour. Each contains a large seed that takes up most of the fruits volume. The fruit itself is grape-like but tougher and has one large seed rather than several small ones. They stay green and hard on the bunch and eventually they change to deep purple colour when mature. They hang in bunches and are about the size of regular grapes.

Culinary Use
When fully mature, they become soft and have a sweet-sour taste. They make great jellies and jams. Sea grapes can make an alcoholic drink similar to wine. They can be eaten raw or cooked and used in salads, soups or sauces.

Nutritional value
Sea grapes contain vitamin A, C, fibre, potassium, calcium, magnesium and iron.

Interesting facts and folklore
The sap has been used for dyeing and tanning leather. A juice made from the plant called Jamaica kino is used to treat dysentery and diarrhoea.

Seville orange
Citrus aurantium

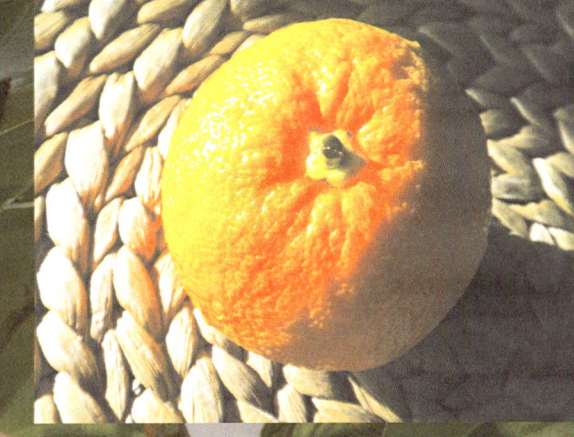

Other names
Bitter orange, bigarade orange, marmalade orange, naranja amarga.

Native habitat
Seville oranges originated in Southeast Asia and spread to the Islamic world by 700 A.D. reaching Spain in the 12th century. They have been growing wild since ancient times by the name "bitter orange".

Description
Seville oranges are typically small to medium-sized, around 7-8 cm in diameter with a yellow-orange rind. The orangey-yellow flesh is filled with seeds and is soft, juicy, and has a sour, acid and slightly bitter taste when ripe.

Culinary Use
Fruit is best juiced as it's very bitter. It has a high pectin content, and is valued for making British orange marmalade. These oranges are harvested once a year in Seville and shipped to Britain for marmalade production due to their excellent setting properties.

Nutritional value
Seville oranges are rich in vitamin C, dietary fibre, and thiamine. They also provide potassium, phosphorus, vitamin A, and calcium.

Interesting facts and folklore
Seville oranges were named from Seville in Spain, where they were introduced from Asia and became a symbol for the city. Seville oranges are thought to be a cross between the pomelo and the mandarin.

Soncoya
Annona purpurea

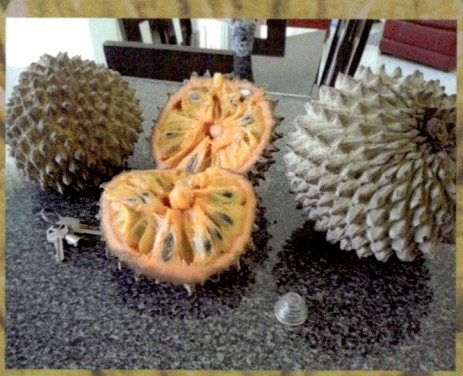

Other names
Soncoya, sincuya, cabeza de negro, yellow ilama, chinkuya, sencuya, and toreta.

Native habitat
Native to the humid forests of Panama, Colombia, Venezuela, to southern Mexico, chiefly at low elevations 400 metres above sea level but sometimes ascending to around 1200 metres above sea level.

Description
Soncoya fruits are round, 12-20 cm wide. They have a hard, spiky skin or shell resembling a durian and short hooks that are curved towards the stem. Pick fruit when the skin changes to a greyish green colour. Fruits are ripe when the stem becomes loose. Slicing it in half with a knife, the skin cuts through with some difficulty. The flesh is a bright orange, creamy with quite a number of seeds. The aromatic ripe fruit has a flavour reminiscent of soursop and tangerine but with a fibrous texture. The tree is mainly grown as a dooryard specimen in its native habitat.

Culinary Use
The pulp is eaten raw or is strained for juice. It can also be used as a garnish on salads. Its stringy texture is best processed through a food mill and made into shakes, smoothies and ice cream. It will keep in the fridge for two weeks.

Nutritional value
This fruit is a great source of vitamins, especially vitamin C. It has potassium, magnesium, and iron.

Interesting facts and folklore
Soncoya juice is used as a remedy for fevers. The inner bark is used for preparing teas, often to treat dysentery.

Soursop
Annona muricata

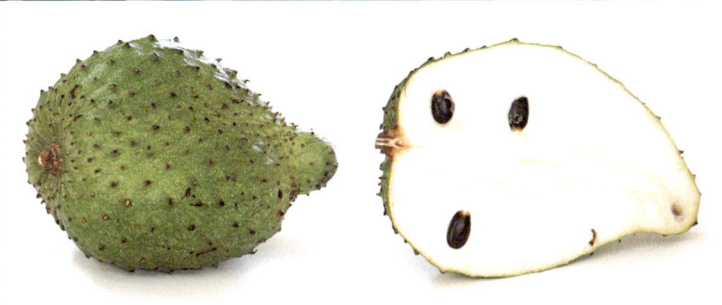

Other names
Guanabana, guyabana sinini, prickly custard apple, durian belanda, graviola, durian europa, durian makkah, durian benggala.

Native habitat
Soursop is native to the tropical regions of the Americas and the Caribbean. Trees prefer lowland areas at altitudes of 0 to 1200 metres (3,900 ft). They cannot stand frost.

Description
Large (up to 30cm long), crooked, roundish or heart shaped fruits with small, soft, fleshy spines. The skin is dark green and turns slightly lighter green when ripe. When ready to eat the fruit is very soft to the touch, and begins to break down quickly. The white flesh is sweet, juicy, and contains large indigestible, black seeds. The flesh is aromatic with a smell like pineapples or bananas, with an acidic flavour. The fruit has a shelf life of only a few days at room temperature.

Culinary Use
The pulp is used to make smoothies, fresh fruit juice, as well as candies, sorbets, and ice cream flavourings. The fresh, meaty flesh is juicy and slightly acid producing a rich and creamy thirst quenching juice. Soursop is delicious when the pulp is pureed with ice-cream.

Nutritional value
Soursop has a significant amount of vitamin C (25-35%) of the daily value, plus good amounts of fibre.

Interesting facts and folklore
Tea brewed from the dried leaves of the soursop tree is used as a sleep aid in the Caribbean. Trees are also the main host plant for tailed jay caterpillars that devour the leaves.

Spanish lime
Melicoccus bijugatis

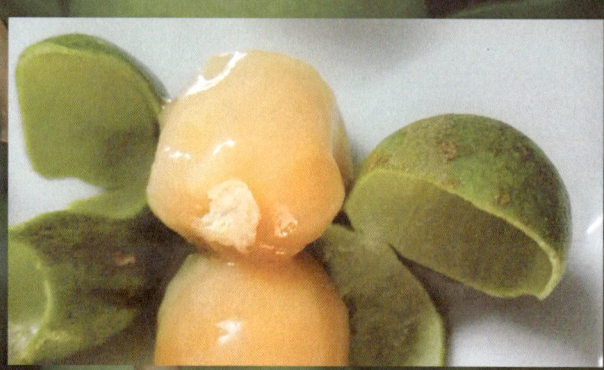

Other names
Quenepa, limoncillo, bajan ackee, mamoncillo, genip, guinep, honey berry.

Native habitat
Spanish limes are native to South America in Venezuela, Brazil, Colombia, and naturalised in coastal and dry forest in Central America, the Caribbean and parts of the Old World tropics.

Description
The fruit is a round stone-bearing fruit, approximately 2–4 cm in diameter, with a thin, brittle, green peel. The bulk of the fruit is made up of the one whitish seed, which is surrounded by an edible, orange, juicy, gelatinous pulp. When ripe, the fruits have a bittersweet, wine-like flavour and have mild laxative properties. The pulp is orange, salmon or yellowish in colour with a somewhat juicy and pasty texture.

Culinary Use
The sweet fruits, which are consumed fresh or canned, and can also be used in the preparation of soft drinks and alcoholic beverages.sweet and gelatinous pulp with a grape-like flavour. eaten out of hand, they can also be cooked in pies, jams and jellies.

Nutritional value
Fruits are extremely rich in iron and phosphorus.

Interesting facts and folklore
In Puerto Rico there is a yearly celebration of Spanish limes known as Festival Nacional de la Quenepa. A decoction of the bark is widely used by local people to treat dysentery. Extracts from the leaves are used in South America to kill flies and repel sandflies and a tea made from young leaves is used in the Dominican Republic to reduce fever.

Strawberry guava
Psidium cattleianum

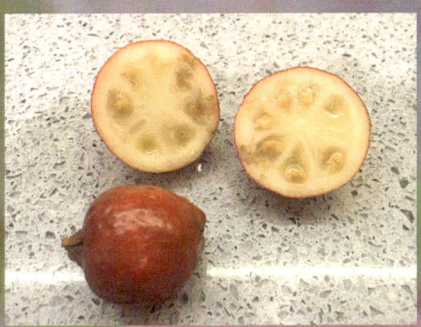

Other names
Cattley guava (this name honours William Cattley, an English horticulturist) cherry guava, Chinese guava, pineapple guava, red guava, red strawberry guava, small guava.

Native habitat
Strawberry guava is home in the Amazonian Basin in Brazil in rainforests up to 1300 metres in elevation.

Description
Strawberry guava fruit is small, yellow to dark red or purple with a thin skin. It is round to oval in shape, and grows to around 2-4 cm long. The yellowish, translucent flesh is both juicy and tart and tastes of wild strawberry. There are many small, brown, edible seeds.

Culinary Use
The whole fruit is usually eaten straight from the tree as the thin skin and the juicy flesh are soft and tasty. They make great jam and juices. Remove the skins for a sweeter flavour. Fruits are commonly used in fruit salads, cakes, and sorbets, but also with salty meat dishes. They have a short shelf life of 2-3 days.

Nutritional value
Strawberry guava contains a flavonoid called hyperoside. This acts as a natural antidepressant, increasing your serotonin levels. Strawberry guava is also rich in vitamin C and potassium.

Interesting facts and folklore
Another common name for the fruit is Cattley guava, named in honour of English horticulturist William Cattley. Necklaces are handcrafted in Tanzania by tying together fruit beads. They are an invasive plant in Hawaii, spread by birds and pigs and have no natural predators. The wood from trees can be burnt to smoke meats.

Sugar apple
Annona squamosa

Other names
Sweetsop, custard apple, anona, nona, sweet apple.

Native habitat
Sweetsop is native to the tropical lowlands of Central America and the Caribbean.

Description
Ripe fruit has segmented flesh that is creamy white to light yellow. They are usually round with a knobbly surface. The sweet and juicy flesh surrounds a brown to black seed. Each fruit has 20 - 40 seeds. Fruit colour is pale green to blue green to red, depending on the variety. The flesh is fragrant and sweet, creamy white through light yellow, and resembles and tastes like custard.

Culinary Use
This delicious, sweet fruit is typically eaten freshly picked or chilled in the refrigerator for 30 minutes. It is used as a dessert or blended into milkshakes, ice cream, and jellies. For a sensational fruit salad serve equal parts sugar apple, strawberries, bananas, and pineapple.

Nutritional value
Sugar apple is an excellent source of vitamin C and manganese, a good source of thiamine and vitamin B6. It also has vitamins B2, B3 B5, B9, iron, magnesium, phosphorus and potassium.

Interesting facts and folklore
In traditional Indian medicine the leaves were crushed for use as a poultice to apply to wounds. In Central America the leaves are put in chicken coops to repel lice.

Tamarillo
Solanum betaceum

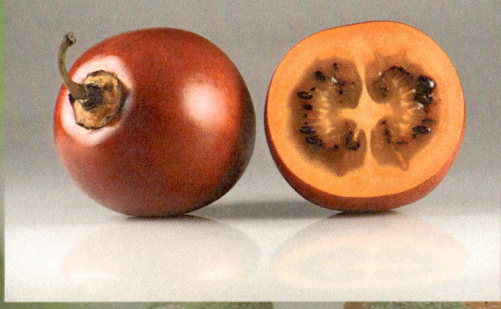

Other names
Tree tomato, tomate de árbol (Spanish), tomate andino, tomate serrano, blood fruit, poor man's tomatoe, terong belanda, Dutch eggplant, tomato-on-a-stick, tomato de castilla.

Native habitat
The tamarillo is native to the Andes of Ecuador, Colombia, Peru, Chile, Argentina and Bolivia. It is a typical fruit of the Andean highlands.

Description
Tamarillo fruits are yellow or red to purple, egg-shaped. Similar to a tomato in texture including the small edible seeds. However in flavour they are sweet like a tomato but with citric, tangy and bitter undertones. The yellow types are generally sweeter and more frequently used in desserts.

Culinary Use
Fruit is eaten raw or cooked. The best varieties are juicy and sub-acid and can be eaten out of hand by cutting the fruit in half and scooping out the flesh. It is often added to fruit salads, or used like tomatoes in salads and sandwiches. More commonly, the unripe tart fruits are used in chutney, curry and hot dishes. Ripe fruits are used in stews, soups, stuffings, cakes, jellies, jams. The fruit contains small, tender, edible seeds. Tamarillo can be mixed into sauces, made into a dessert topping, juiced and also pickled.

Nutritional value
Tamarillo has vitamin A, C, and is rich in vitamin E, provitamin A, potassium and iron.

Interesting facts and folklore
Warmed leaves are wrapped around the neck as a remedy for sore throat. Tamarillo is closely related to other Solanaceae members of vegetables and fruits such as tomato, eggplant, and chilli peppers.

Umbu
Spondias tuberosa

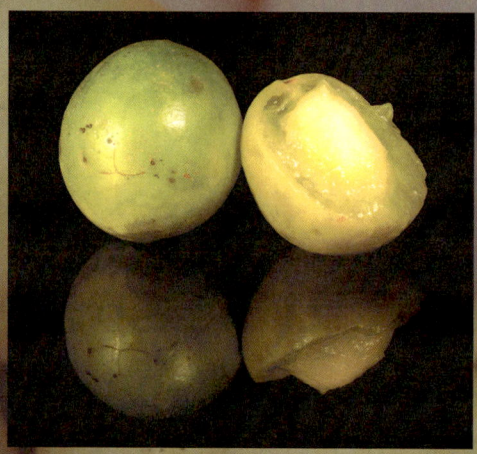

Other names
Imbu, Brazil plum.

Native habitat
Umbu is home to the dry plains and scrublands of northeastern Brazil. It grows in the Caatinga forest where the climate is hot and dry for months.

Description
The Umbu is a small, round fruit (2-4 cm), light yellow to red in colour with a smooth, leathery shell or peel. The flesh is soft, juicy, and melting with a sweet-tart taste and smell. Umbu fruits are green or yellow when ripe, and their flesh has a large seed.

Culinary Use
Umbu are eaten fresh or made into jams and preserved. It is the base of a vinagre (the juice pressed from overripe fruit) mixed with sugar and milk to make *imbuzada*, a drink from northeastern Brazil, and it is especially popular in Bahia. A jam can be made by pressing together layers of dried umbu paste.

Nutritional value
Umbu contains vitamins A, B1, B2, and C and the minerals calcium, iron and phosphorus.

Interesting facts and folklore
The name of this tree and fruit comes from the indigenous phrase y-mb-u, which means *tree that gives drink*. Its roots store starch and water in storage organs known as "tuberous aquifers".

Velvet Tamarind
Dialium cochinchinense

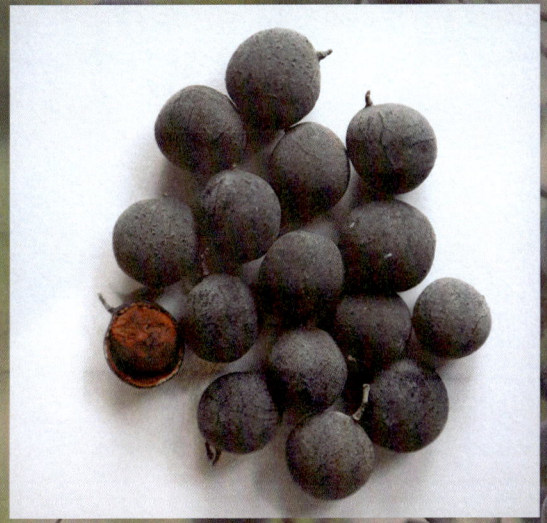

Other names
Keranji, Sierra Leone-tamarind, West African velvet tamarind.

Native habitat
Velvet tamarind is native to Borneo, Cambodia, Laos, Malaya, Thailand, Vietnam.

Description
This medium-sized, deciduous tree is widely distributed in lowland forests to 800 m in Southeast Asia. It is popular for its velvety, blackish fruits that have a sweet pulp similar to tamarind and its dense, hardwood traded as Keranji.

Culinary Use
Fruit has an edible sweet pulp, similar to tamarind but not as tasty. Ripened fruits can be mixed with sugar and chilli peppers and sold as dessert. Alternatively, the fruit can be dried until the skin cracks open and the brown pulp is visible, ensuring thorough drying for preservation. The pulp, along with seeds, is then separated from the rind by shaking it.

Nutritional value
Pulp of the fruit is rich in vitamin C, sodium, iron, magnesium and potassium.

Interesting facts and folklore
Fruit has diverse medical applications, including treating gastric ulcers, hypertension, bronchitis, diabetes, menstrual pains, and wound healing.

Wampee
Clausena lansium

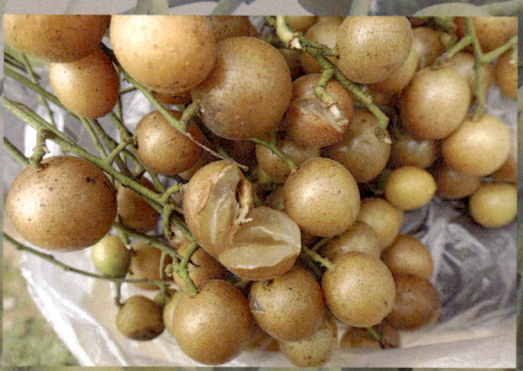

Other names
Fool's curry leaf, wampi, uampi, hong bi. wanpi or huang pi ("yellow skin" in Mandarin).

Native habitat
Wampee is a distant relative of the citrus fruits and is native to southern China and the northern and central provinces of Vietnam. The tree is subtropical to tropical, and tolerant of light frosts. They grow in a wide range of soils, including deep sand and limestone soils, but prefer well drained, sandy loam soils.

Description
Wampee fruits are grape-sized, round and aromatic. They can range from sweet to tangy or slightly sour, depending on the variety. When ripe, wampee fruits turn brownish-yellow and have a thin, brittle skin resembling paper. They typically contain 1-2 seeds per fruit and are best left to ripen fully on the tree for best flavour. The flavour is a delightful blend of sweet and tangy, reminiscent of grape, lychee, and citrus.

Culinary Use
Wampees are sweet and sugary, with a pleasant sourness. Use freshly picked berries with ice cream, chocolates, and other fruits. Wampee fruit is eaten raw, but also cooked with meats, or in other dishes for the sweet/sour flavour. Wampee can also be found dried, preserved as jams, pickled, and in soups.

Nutritional value
Wampee is low in calories and fat. Very high in vitamin C, and a good source of vitamin B3.

Interesting facts and folklore
The wampee has been used to treat a wide range of health issues such as tooth decay, postpartum concerns, headaches, dyspepsia, and intestinal worms.

Yellow mombin
Spondias mombin

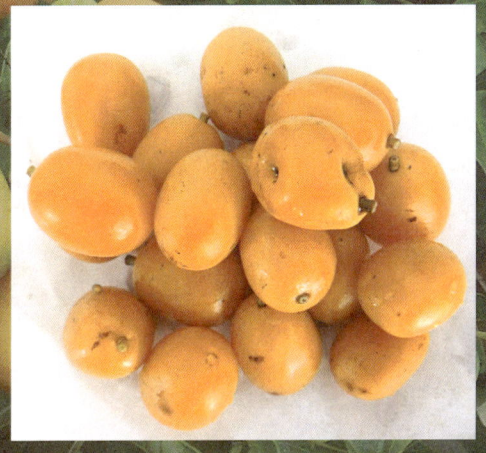

Other names
Jobo, hog plum, Jamaica plum, cajá-mirim, taperebá, tepereba, nkunia guenguere kunansieto, imbu, ubos, mango ciruelo, prunier mombi.

Native habitat
Yellow mombin is native to the tropical Americas, including the West Indies. They grow best in the subhumid and frost-free tropics, where they can be found at elevations up to 1,000 metres above sea level.

Description
Yellow mombin is a light orange to yellow or brown fruit. There is a lot of variation in fruit quality, some being sweet and pleasant and others quite disagreeable. The crunchy pulp tastes like a mix between pineapple and mango.

Culinary Use
Fruit is eaten raw or cooked with sugar, jams, and ice cream. It is also steamed and eaten as a vegetable with salted fish and rice.

Nutritional value
Fruits contain a considerable amount of pro-vitamin A and a portion of the pulp can provide up to one third of the recommended daily allowance of vitamin A. They have good antioxidant activity and significant amounts of fibre, phenolic compounds, carotenoids, vitamin C, and minerals.

Interesting fact and folklore
Water from the roots of this tree can be drunk when other supplies run out. Yellow mombin is stewed and given to treat diarrhoea.

Photo Credits

The photographers maintain copyright to all photos. No photos may be reproduced without the express written consent of the photographers.

Front cover: Rambutans, Deepugn/WikimediaCommins

Back cover: Canistel (fruit), wasanajai/Shutterstock

Title page: Abyssinian dovyalis (2), robert gibson z/Shutterstock

Index pages: (Amazon), Neil Palmer/CIAT/WikimediaCommons

About the author page : Amazon rainforest in Tena, Ecuador, ihttps://www.flickr.com/photos/jaybock / WikimediaCommons

Introduction: Rare fruit plant and seed hunter, Alan Carle www.botanicalark.com; Banjarmasin floating market, Mahfud651 / WikimediaCommons;
(Rainforest), Shao/WikimediaCommons

Photo credits pages: (Amazon), jlwad/WikimediaCommons

Abiu (2), Forest and Kim Starr/WikimediaCommons

Abyssinian dovyalis (2), robert gibson z/Shutterstock

Acai palm (tree fruit), JULIO CESAR BALDIM/WikimediaCommons; (fruit) PARALAXIS/Shutterstock

Acerola (tree fruit), Zaiane Sá/WikimediaCommons; (fruit)Túllio F /WikimediaCommons

Ackee (tree fruit),Saliousoft /WikimediaCommons; (fruit) Ralf Steinberger/WikimediaCommons

Amazon tree grape (tree fruit), Kristof Zyskowski & Yulia Bereshpolova/WikimediaCommons;
(fruit) guentermanaus/Shutterstock

Ambarella (tree fruit), Prenn/WikimediaCommons;
(fruit)Paulo Vilela /Shutterstock

Araza (fruit extraction),EditorDoro /WikimediaCommons;
(fruit) Jack7_7/Shutterstock

Atemoya (tree fruit),AJCespedes /Shutterstock;
(fruit) Vladirina32 / Shutterstock

Avocado (tree fruit),Kondah /WikimediaCommons;
(fruit) Formulatehealth/WikimediaCommons

Bael fruit (tree fruit),FON's Fasai /Shutterstock; (fruit)
Asit K GoshThaumaturgist/WikimediaCommons

Bakupari (tree fruit and fruit),Alex Popovkin, Bahia, Brazil /
WikimediaCommons; Nino Bautz / Shutterstock

Barbados gooseberry (tree fruit), Nadiatalent/
WikimediaCommons; (fruit) Mario Andrioli/Shutterstock

Bignay (tree fruit), MarvinBikolano/WikimediaCommons;
(fruit) Fitri Chairiyah/Shutterstock

Bilimbi (tree fruit), Mullookkaaran/WikimediaCommons;
(fruit) Creatifood/Shutterstock

Black sapote (tree fruit), Yonathon Galler/WikimediaCommons;
(fruit) KATHERINE WAGNER-REISS/WikimediaCommons

Borojo (tree fruit), Elminafaz/Shutterstock;
(fruit) Barna Tanko/Shutterstock

Breadfruit (tree fruit),Forest and Kim Starr /
WikimediaCommons; (fruit) Kgbo/WikimediaCommons

Bullocks heart (tree fruit), Sridhar Rao/
WikimediaCommons; (fruit) anny ta/Shutterstock

Burdekin plum (tree & fruit),Steve Fitzgerald /WikimediaCommins

Caimito (fruit in hand), Forest and Kim Starr/
WikimediaCommons; (fruit) wasanajai/Shutterstock

Camu camu (tree fruit),Túllio F /WikimediaCommins;
(fruit) Juan Carlos QM /Shutterstock

Canistel (tree fruit), Forest and Kim Starr/
WikimediaCommons; (fruit) wasanajai/Shutterstock

Carambola (tree fruit), Mailamal/WikimediaCommons;
(fruit) nine_far / shutterstock

Cashew apple (tree fruit), Abhishek Jacob/WikimediaCommons;
(fruit) Dr. Raju Kasambe/WikimediaCommons

Cecropia (tree fruit),Casa Comum Terra/shutterstock;
(fruit) NANCY AYUMI KUNIHIRO/Shutterstock

Ceylon gooseberry (tree fruit), DRSHAGGY151/
WikimediaCommons; (fruit) Alexandre Laprise/Shutterstock

Cherimoya (tree fruit), SAplants/WikimediaCommons;
(fruit) Tgdileep/WikimediaCommons

Chinese jujube (fruit in hand),תימס-ןיקלג הזילע /
WikimediaCommons; (fruit) GWX / shutterstock

Coco plum (tree fruit), Filo gèn'/WikimediaCommons; (fruit
in hand)Forest and Kim Starr /WikimediaCommons

Cocona (fruit),guentermanaus /Shutterstock;
(fruit) Dtarazona/WikimediaCommons

Coconut (tree fruit),കാക്കര /WikimediaCommons;
(fruit) Ivar Leidus/WikimediaCommons

Common guava (tree fruit),Kwameghana(Bright Kwame Ayisi)
/WikimediaCommons; (fruit) miniartkur /shutterstock

Cuban mangosteen (fruit), www.TopTropicals.
com / WikimediaCommons

Dabai (fruit), Nora Yusuf/Shutterstock

Date (tree fruit), ImagePerson/WikimediaCommons;
(fruit) Ogalihillary/WikimediaCommons

Downy rose cherry (tree fruit),Forest and Kim Starr / WikimediaCommons; (fruit) Mokkie/WikimediaCommons

Durian (tree fruit), AmonHeijne/WikimediaCommons; (fruit) Rod Waddington/WikimediaCommons

Gamboge (tree fruit), Dinesh Valke/WikimediaCommons; (fruit) Forest and Kim Starr / WikimediaCommons;

Giant granadilla (tree fruit), Frankguillen/WikimediaCommons; (fruit) Mabelin Santos/Shutterstock

Green sapote , (fruit) I Like Plants!/WikimediaCommons

Guavaberry (fruit),Ymleon /WikimediaCommons
; www.guavaberry.com

Herbert River cherry (fruit),Judgefloro /WikimediaCommons

Ilama (tree fruit), I Like Plants!/WikimediaCommons; (fruit) Edgar p miller/WikimediaCommons

Imbe (tree), Ton Rulkens/WikimediaCommons; (tree fruit) Christopher Hind/WikimediaCommons

Indian gooseberry (tree fruit), A. J. T. Johnsingh, WWF-India and NCF/WikimediaCommons; (fruit) Yosri/WikimediaCommons

Inga (tree fruit and fruit), Burkhard Mücke/WikimediaCommons

Jaboticaba (tree fruit), Bruno.karklis/ WikimediaCommons; (fruit) Forest and Kim Starr/WikimediaCommons

Jackfruit (tree fruit),无情介壳虫 /WikimediaCommons; (fruit) Biswarup Ganguly/WikimediaCommons

Jelly palm (tree fruit),Moxfyre /WikimediaCommons; (fruit) Forest and Kim Starr/WikimediaCommons

Kaffir plum (tree fruit), SAplants/WikimediaCommons

Karonda (tree fruit), Sakurai Midori/WikimediaCommons; Michael Hermann, http://www.cropsforthefuture.org/WikimediaCommons

Kei apple (tree fruit), SAplants/WikimediaCommons; (fruit) vainillaychile/ Shutterstock

Key lime (tree fruit), Forest and Kim Starr/WikimediaCommons; (fruit) T Voekler/WikimediaCommons

Kiwifruit (tree fruit), Zeynel Cebeci/WikimediaCommons; (fruit) Theo Crazzolara/WikimediaCommons

Kwai muk (tree fruit), Forest and Kim Starr/WikimediaCommons; (fruit) www.daleysfruit.com.au

Langsat (tree fruit), Len Worthington/WikimediaCommons; (fruit) Judgefloro/WikimediaCommons

Lucuma (tree fruit), lovelypeace / Shutterstock; (fruit) Ildi Papp / Shutterstock

Mabolo (tree fruit),Rison Thumboor /WikimediaCommons; (fruit) Forest and Kim Starr/WikimediaCommons

Madrono (tree fruit),Umberto Ferrando/WikimediaCommons; (fruit) Camera.Winy / shutterstock

Malay apple (tree fruit), Forest and Kim Starr/WikimediaCommons; Dhemen Studio/shutterstock

Mamey sapote (tree fruit), Peggy GrebImage Number D965-1/WikimediaCommons; (fruit) Sharon Hahn Darlin/WikimediaCommons

Mangaba (tree fruit), Tarciso Leão/WikimediaCommons; (fruit) Cacio Murilo/shutterstock

Mango (tree fruit),Dinesh Valke /WikimediaCommons; (fruit)Ivar Leidus / WikimediaCommons

Mangosteen (tree fruit), VpuipV/WikimediaCommons; (fruit)Basile Morin /WikimediaCommons

Maprang (tree fruit), Mattis/WikimediaCommons; (fruit) wasanajai/Shutterstock

Matisia (tree fruit), Luis Echeverri Urrea / Shutterstock; (fruit) Xemenendura /WikimediaCommons

Maqui berry (tree fruit), Denis.prévôt/WikimediaCommons; (fruit) Hector Montero/WikimediaCommons

Miracle fruit (tree fruit), V C Balakrishnan /WikimediaCommons; (fruit) Forest and Kim Starr /WikimediaCommons

Mountain soursop (tree fruit), F. Inushita /shutterstock; (fruit); Jobz Fotografia / shutterstock

Nance fruit (fruit), Koffermejia/WikimediaCommons; (fruit) Byron Sagastume/shutterstock

Naranjilla (tree fruit), Hector Montero /WikimediaCommons; (fruit) Veryhuman/WikimediaCommons

Otaheite gooseberry (tree fruit and fruit), PJeganathan/WikimediaCommons

Panama berry (tree fruit), Vinayaraj /WikimediaCommons; (fruit) Roby Nurhidayat / Shutterstock

Papaya (tree fruit), H. Zell / WikimediaCommons; (fruit) Forest and Kim Starr/WikimediaCommons

Passionfruit (vine fruit), Forest and Kim Starr /WikimediaCommons; (fruit) Alexander Klink /WikimediaCommons

Peach palm (fruit), Michael Hermann/WikimediaCommons; (fruit) David Yela/WikimediaCommons

Persimmon (tree fruit), Vinayaraj /WikimediaCommons; (fruit) Frank Schulenburg/WikimediaCommons

Pitaya (tree fruit), Bùi Thuy Đào Nguyên/WikimediaCommons; (fruit) Rodrigo.Argenton/WikimediaCommons

Pomegranate (tree fruit), azerbaijan_ stockers/ Shutterstock; (fruit) Ivar Leidus/WikimediaCommons

Pomelo (tree fruit), Agnieszka Kwiecień, Nova/
WikimediaCommons; (fruit) Ivar Leidus/WikimediaCommons

Prickly pear (tree fruit), Tomás Castelazo/WikimediaCommons;
(fruit) Karen and Brad Emerson/WikimediaCommons

Pulasan (tree fruit), Norman Ong/Shutterstock;
(fruit) sasirin pamai/Shutterstock

Rambai (tree fruit), RAP21/Shutterstock;
(fruit) Satsuei_athian/Shutterstock

Rambutan (tree fruit), Rison Thumboor/WikimediaCommons;
(fruit) Ivar Leidus/WikimediaCommons

Red mombin (tree fruit), Forest and Kim Starr/
WikimediaCommons; (fruit) mircea dobre / Shutterstock

Rollinia (tree fruit); Jack7_7/shutterstock;
(fruit) guentermanaus/Shutterstock

Santol (fruits), Judgefloro/WikimediaCommons

Sapodilla (tree fruit), Rison Thumboor/WikimediaCommons;
(fruit) Nungning20/Shutterstock

Sea grape (tree fruit), Wilfredor/WikimediaCommons;
(fruit) Jody Ann/Shutterstock

Seville orange (tree fruit), Zeynel Cebeci/WikimediaCommons;
(fruit) Amanda Slater/WikimediaCommons

Soncoya (tree fruit), Ll1324/WikimediaCommons;
(fruit) Raulglezruiz https://tropicalfruitforum.com/
index.php?topic=25676.0 Tropical fruit forum

Soursop (tree fruit), Wong Gunkid /Shutterstock; (fruit)
Muhammad Mahdi Karim/WikimediaCommons

Spanish lime (tree fruit, fruit), Filo gèn'/WikimediaCommons;
Alvaro de J. Carcaño Loeza /WikimediaCommons

Strawberry guava (tree fruit), Agnieszka Kwiecień, Nova/WikimediaCommons; (fruit) Yonygg/WikimediaCommons

Sugar apple (tree fruit), Vengolis / WikimediaCommons; (fruit) Kristof Zyskowski & Yulia Bereshpolova /WikimediaCommons

Tamarillo (tree fruit),Sridhar Rao /WikimediaCommons; (fruit)Ivar Leidus /WikimediaCommons

Tamarind (tree fruit), Tau'olunga/WikimediaCommons; (fruit) Ivar Leidus/WikimediaCommons

Umbu (fruit),renatamomo / Shutterstock; (fruit) Rodrigo.Argenton/WikimediaCommons

Velvet tamarind (tree fruit), Apinya Anphanlam/Shutterstock; (fruit) Ezagren/WikimediaCommons

Wampee (tree fruit)Anna Frodesiak, /WikimediaCommons; (fruit) SIRIMAT KAMSAIIN/Shutterstock

Yellow jaboticaba (tree fruit), Daniela Branco/WikimediaCommons; (fruit) www.daleysfruit.com.au

Yellow mombin (tree fruit), Filo gèn'/WikimediaCommons; (fruit) Adoscam/WikimediaCommons

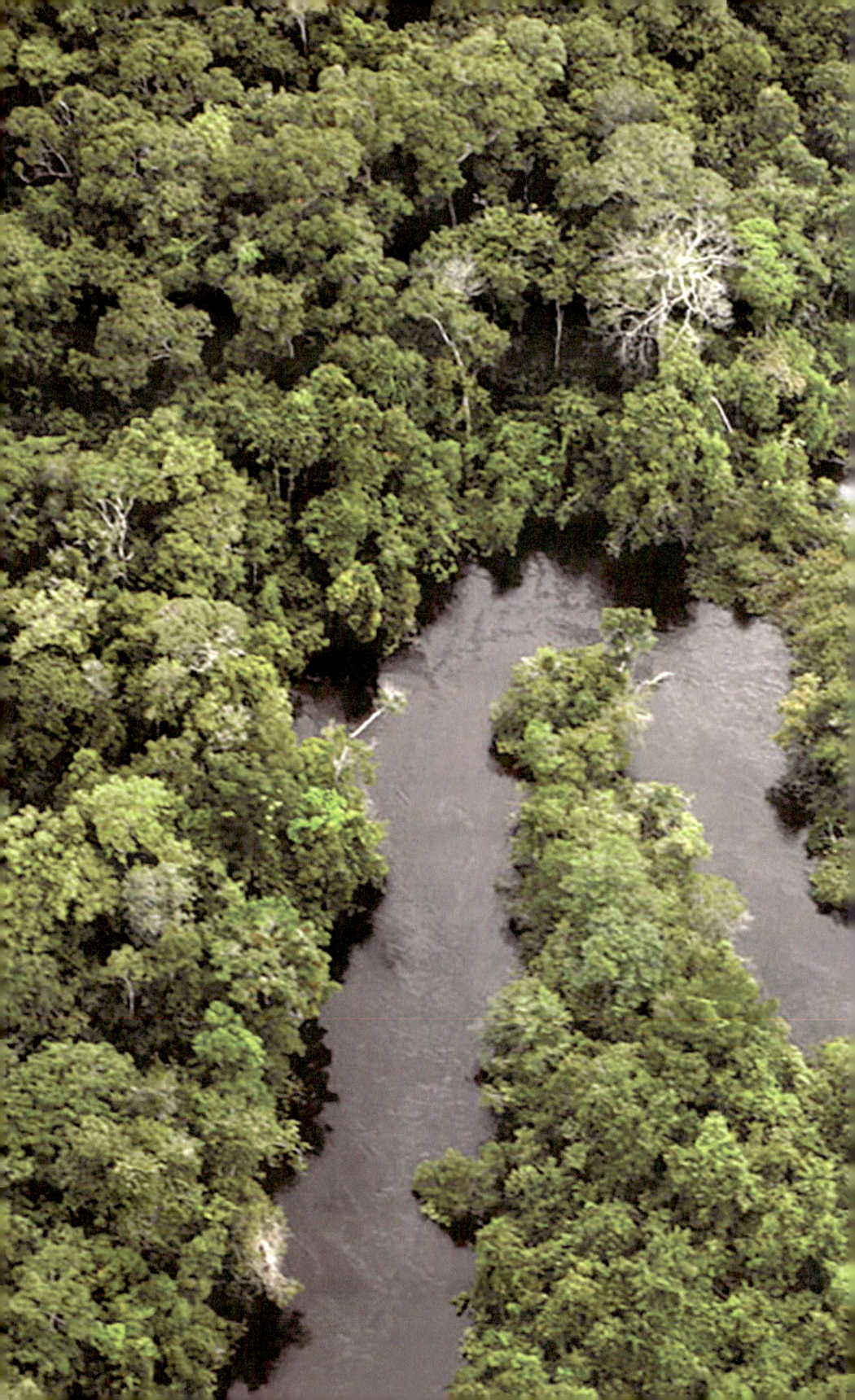

www.ingramcontent.com/pod-product-compliance
Lightning Source LLC
Chambersburg PA
CBRC091504220426
43661CB00051B/1552